THE PREPARATION OF SOLUTIONS ISOOSMOTIC WITH BLOOD, TEARS, AND TISSUE

CONTRIBUTIONS FROM THE DANISH PHARMACOPOEIA COMMISSION

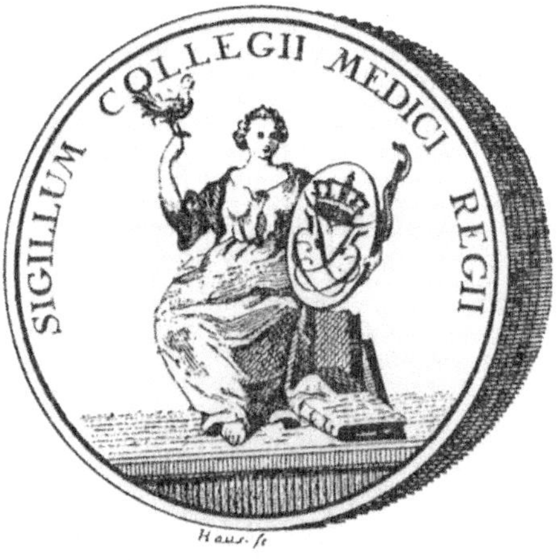

VOL. II

THE PREPARATION OF SOLUTIONS ISOOSMOTIC WITH BLOOD, TEARS, AND TISSUE

1947

EINAR MUNKSGAARD
PUBLISHER
COPENHAGEN

HEINEMANN
MEDICAL BOOKS · LTD.
LONDON

THE PREPARATION OF SOLUTIONS ISOOSMOTIC WITH BLOOD, TEARS, AND TISSUE

BY

C. G. Lund, E. Peülicke Nielsen and K. Pedersen-Bjergaard

1947

EINAR MUNKSGAARD
PUBLISHER
COPENHAGEN

HEINEMANN
MEDICAL BOOKS · LTD.
LONDON

FIRST PUBLISHED 1947

PRINTED IN DENMARK
BY
H. P. HANSENS BOGTRYKKERI
COPENHAGEN

FROM THE DISPENSARY OF
BISPEBJERG HOSPITAL
COPENHAGEN

CHIEF:
K. Pedersen-Bjergaard Ph. D.

PREFACE

During the work on the new edition of the Danish Pharmacopoeia, it very soon became evident that the question of the correct osmotic concentration in liquids for instillation into the conjunctiva could hardly be answered on the basis of the literature concerning this subject, a literature which seems to be characterized more by tradition than by experience based on experiments. So it was decided to submit the problem to a closer examination, and in addition to examine the possibility of arriving at such prescriptions as would allow of the preparation of other eyedrops than the official ones, so as to give them the correct osmotic concentration. When this proved to be possible, the work was extended so as to include solutions for injection, both official and non-official ones.

By using the curves in the present work it will be possible to prepare isotonic solutions of a large number of the commonly employed remedies in therapeutics, both for injection and for application to the eyes. They enable the pharmacist to prepare extemporaneously described fluids of the correct osmotic concentration, and it is the hope of the Commission that this paper may also be of value to the work in other pharmaceutical laboratories in Denmark, and abroad.

Copenhagen, January 15th, 1947.

KNUD O. MØLLER,
Chairman of the Danish
Pharmacopoeia Commission.

TRANSLATED INTO ENGLISH

BY

Hans Tang

CONTENTS

ACKNOWLEDGMENTS

In the summer of 1939 the Chairman of the Danish Pharmacopoeia Commission, Professor *K. O. Møller,* M. D., Director of the University Institute of Pharmacology, Copenhagen, expressed his desire that the Pharmacy Committee of the Commission should prepare the rules for official preparation of eye drops, isotonic with lachrymal fluid, for the coming edition of the Danish Pharmacopoeia. Professor Møller has, however, not only formulated the task, but he has followed the progression of the work with a constant and keen interest, as gradually it was extended to cover substances that are used in injection therapy, and for local treatment of tissues, where it is also important to prepare isotonic solutions. I shall always remember Professor Møller's encouragement and initiative with pleasure and gratitude; they have been a very good support to me in the accomplishment of this task.

The Chairman of the Pharmacy Committee in the Pharmacopoeia Commission, Professor *S. Aa. Schou,* Ph. D., Sc. D., Chief of the Dispensary of the State Hospital, Copenhagen, entrusted the solution of this task to me, and I want to thank Professor Schou, and my two other colleagues in the Pharmacy Committee, Apoteker *E. Høst-Madsen,* Ph. D., and *Kaj Nielsen,* cand. pharm., for the interest they have shown me, and the assistance they have given me.

The determination of the freezing point depressions were carried out at the Dispensary of Bispebjerg Hospital, whereas the numerous vapour pressure determinations were made at the University Laboratory of Zoophysiology, Copenhagen. Both the former director of the laboratory, Professor *August Krogh,* Ph. D., M. D., L. L. D., Sc. D., and its present director, Professor *P. Brandt Rehberg,* Ph. D., have shown us the greatest hospitality and helpfulness. Thus it was in collaboration with Professor Krogh that we succeeded in showing that lachrymal fluid has the same osmotic pressure as blood. The Assistant at the University Laboratory of Zoophysiology, *Hans Ussing,* Ph. D., has helped us with much instruction, good advice, and criticism. I want very much to express my best thanks to Professor Krogh, Professor Brandt Rehberg, and Dr. Ussing for the unselfish way in which they have always lent us a helping hand in our work at the University Laboratory of Zoophysiology.

Professor *H. Berry,* B. Sc., Ph. C., F. R. J. C., Dip. Bact., Dean at the college of the Pharmaceutical Society, University of London, and his Assistant, Mr. *D. Train,* B. Pharm., have rendered us great service in reading through our work, and have helped us with their good advice, also in reading the English translation for us, and we want to express our deepest appreciation of their kindness in doing so.

In the calculation of the error in the vapour pressure determinations, valuable assistance was given us by Lektor *G. Rasch,* Ph. D.

Adjunkt *Hans Tang,* cand. mag., who has translated the work into English, has often given me valuable advice, and I would thank him for the care and interest he has expended on the translation.

Laboratory Assistant, *C. C. Jensen,* cand. phil., and Mr. *Keld Pedersen* have made the extensive draftman's work in a most satisfactory manner.

Finally I want to expres my thanks to the Danish Home Office and the National Health Service, which made the publication of the work possible, through economical support from »Apotekerfonden«.

It would not have been possible to carry through the comprehensive experimental work in such a short time (1940—1945) without the valuable cooperation of two of the assistants attached to the Dispensary of Bispebjerg Hospital, *E. Peülicke Nielsen,* cand. pharm. (1940—41), and *C. G. Lund,* cand. pharm. (1942—1945). I hereby give them my deepfelt thanks for 6 years of faithful and unforgettable cooperation.

The Dispensary of Bispebjerg Hospital,
Copenhagen, January 1947.

KAJ PEDERSEN-BJERGAARD,
Ph. D.

I. INTRODUCTION

The chairman of the Danish Pharmacopoeia Commission, Professor K. O. Møller, M. D., Director of the University Institute of Pharmacology, Copenhagen, has pointed out the need for data to establish rules in the formulation of extemporaneous isoosmotic eye preparations for use in the new Danish Pharmacopoeia. In this paper we have attempted to supply this information as a result of a large number of freezing point and vapour pressure determinations of solutions of appropriate drugs. From the data obtained, we have made proposals for the correction of prescriptions relating to eye preparations in the Dispensatorium Danicum, and have also shown how isoosmotic solutions can easily be obtained for extemporaneous preparations in general.

Furthermore we have carefully checked the existing freezing point and vapour pressure determinations of a number of substances that are used in the preparation of solutions for parenteral injections and solutions for local treatment of tissues, and we have also made determinations of a number of substances that are generally used for the above mentioned purposes, and of which we have found no results stated in literature.

The results have been shown in corresponding tables and curves for practical use.

The freezing point determinations have been made at the Dispensary of Bispebjerg Hospital, Copenhagen.

The vapour pressure determinations have been made in the University Laboratory of Zoophysiology, Copenhagen.

II. OSMOTIC PRESSURE, VAPOUR PRESSURE, BOILING POINT ELEVATION, AND FREEZING POINT DEPRESSION

The first of the methods that have been used for the determination of the osmotic pressure was described in 1882 by *de Vries* who watched the plasmolysis of plant cells in hypertonic solutions.

Then *Hamburger* in 1883 introduced the hæmolytic method, which is based on the principle that the volume of the corpuscles depend on the osmotic pressure of the surrounding fluid, and that two saline solutions that convey the same volume to the same number of corpuscles are isotonic. Since then the use of the changes in weight that take place in tissues immersed in different saline solutions has been tried as a measure of the osmotic pressure. Far greater accuracy, however, is obtained by using the physical methods of determination, but before we go into a detailed description of a few of these, the theoretical background of the osmotic pressure of solutions will be briefly mentioned.

As is well known, the ideal gas equation, according to *van't Hoff*, holds good also for ideal solutions. The equation of the ideal gases is

$$p \cdot v = n \cdot R \cdot T$$

p being the pressure of the gas, v the volume of the gas, n the number of molecules, R the gas constant, and T the absolute temperature. In the case of ideal solutions, the osmotic pressure of the solution, P, replaces the pressure of the gas, p, and the volume of the solution, V, replaces the volume of the gas, v. Thus we have

$$P \cdot V = n \cdot R \cdot T$$

As V is the number of litres of the solution in question, and n the number of un-ionized molecules, n/V equals the molarity of the solution, C, so the formula becomes:

$$P = C \cdot R \cdot T$$

From this formula it is evident that un-ionized solutions of the same molar concentration must have the same osmotic pressure at the same temperature. Such solutions are called isoosmotic. If the dissolved substance is dissociated, the osmotic pressure will increase correspondingly, since it is the concentration of all the particles of the solution that matters.

Thus the osmotic pressure of solutions containing several substances can be found by addition of the pressures that each of the components would have exercised.

In this place it is natural to mention a physiological fact which might be of importance at the preparation of some types of eye drops. This is illustrated by some experiments, quoted from *Heilbrunn (1937)*, made with eggs of the sea-urchin (Echinus). Determined by means of the freezing point depression a 0.53 molar solution of sodium chloride had proved to be isoosmotic with sea-water. This agreed with the fact that the eggs neither shrink nor swell in this saline solution. Based on freezing point determinations a 0.37 molar solution of calcium chloride was also found to be isoosmotic with sea-water. In spite of this, however, the eggs shrank considerably when placed in this solution. By experiments it was found that a 0.29 molar solution of calcium chloride must be used to avoid shrinkage as well as swelling. Solutions that by physical and chemical determinations show the same freezing point, boiling point, vapour pressure, osmotic pressure, etc. are isoosmotic, but, as has been shown in the above example, they need not be isotonic to a given membrane; there are such membranes, which have specific permeability relations to certain substances.

»In actual practice, whenever possible, it is advisable to determine the isotonic concentration of a given solution for the cells on which it is to be used. Often this is not practicable, and it is then customary to use solutions which are believed to be isotonic on the basis of calculation or freezing point determination«. *(Heilbrunn (1937))*.

So it is not improbable that special investigations concerning the permeability of the cornea to the substances that are generally used in eye drops, would reveal similar conditions. Therefore, in the present treatise we have carefully avoided using the expression »tear-isotonicity«, because we have made no determinations directly on the eye.

Sandell (1945) warns against too rigid an application of physical and chemical methods of determination for calculating the isotonicity of solutions for injection. Thus Sandell mentions that aqueous solutions of boric acid, hexamethylentetramine, urethane, and urea, although physically and chemically isotonic, cause hæmolysis when red corpuscles are admixed with them, because solutions of these substances very quickly pass through the membrane of the cell. So he proposes that in the preparation of isotonic solutions no consideration at all should be taken to the part these four substances play in forming the osmotic pressure of solutions. As against this, *Steiger (1945)* proposes that the method of hæmolysis is quite impracticable for the determination of the isotonicity of substances, since several substances, as boric acid and saponin cause hæmolysis, quite irrespective of the concentration.

If the task is to prepare a solution of a substance so that it becomes isotonic with blood, and the osmotic pressure of the solution has been found physically, it must be ascertained if the osmotic pressure is effective or not to the given membrane, in the present case that of the red blood-cell. This depends first and foremost on the lipoid solubility. If the latter is great, the substance will, even in an aqueous solution, penetrate the lipoid membrane of the corpuscles, and cause hæmolysis. So it is not the absolute, but the effective osmotic pressure which one must know in order to prepare a solution that is isotonic with a liquid surrounded by a permeable membrane. Fortunately the effective osmotic pressures of most of the substances with which we have been concerned are of the same magnitude as that of the absolute osmotic pressure. Three of the substances, however, that we have examined, form exceptions because of their fairly good lipoid solubility, namely boric acid, hexamethylentetramine, and urethane.

In the same way that the osmotic pressure of a solution increases proportionally, so the vapour pressure of the solution decreases proportionally with a rising concentration. Thus, determinations of the osmotic pressure can be made, not only directly by determination in an osmometer, but also indirectly by determination of the vapour pressure.

Among other methods for the determination of the osmotic pressure of solutions, the following two are much used: the determination of the boiling point elevation, and especially the determination of the freezing point depression.

The boiling point elevation and the freezing point depression are both proportional to the osmolar concentration. In this paper only freezing point depression is mentioned in detail. It follows *Raoult*'s law which can be expressed by the following equation:

$$t = \frac{k \cdot g \cdot 1000}{M \cdot L} \qquad (I)$$

t being the freezing point depression that the solution shows in relation to the solvent, k the molar freezing point depression of the solvent, g the weight (expressed in grammes) of the dissolved substance, M the molecular weight of the dissolved substance, and L the total weight of the solvent and the substance. Naturally *Raoul's* law is only in force if the substance and the solvent do not react chemically with each other, and moreover the law is only in force in the case of dilute solutions.

If now by means of equation I it is required to prepare solutions which are to be isoosmotic with blood serum the freezing point depression of blood serum (0.56^0) is inserted into the equation instead of t, and the molar freezing point depression of water (1.86^0) instead of k. If it is required to prepare for instance 1000 cubic centimetres of a solution of sucrose ($M = 342$), the concentration is found by means of equation I:

$$0.56 = \frac{1.86 \cdot g \cdot 1000}{342 \cdot 1000}$$

$$g = \frac{0.56 \cdot 342}{1.86} = 103$$

and that is to say that a 10.3 % w/v solution of sucrose is isoosmotic with blood serum. If, however, the substance in question is dissociated in an aqueous solution, the number of ions must be taken into consideration. In the case of sodium chloride this may be represented by

$$NaCl = Na^+ + Cl^-,$$

and in the case of sodium sulphate this may be represented by

$$Na_2SO_4 = 2\ Na^+ + SO_4^{--},$$

i. e. that the freezing point depression of sodium chloride is about twice greater and of sodium sulphate about three times greater than calculated by means of equation I.

In such cases the following equation is employed

$$t = \frac{n \cdot k \cdot g \cdot 1000}{M \cdot L} \qquad (II)$$

where n denotes the number of ions in which the substance is dissociated. For instance if 1000 cubic centimetres of a sodium chloride solution ($M = 58.46$) are to be prepared, the concentration by means of equation II is

$$0.56 = \frac{2 \cdot 1.86 \cdot g \cdot 1000}{58.46 \cdot 1000}$$

$$g = \frac{0.56 \cdot 58.46}{2 \cdot 1.86} = 8.8$$

i. e. that a sodium chloride solution of 0.88 % w/v is isoosmotic with blood serum. The latter method of calculation will, however, only be correct if it is a case of a much diluted solution. In more concentrated solutions the forces at work among the ions themselves have the effect that the osmotic pressure does not become quite so great as should have been expected from the number of ions. The calculated concentration therefore ought to be corrected through division by a factor f (the activity coefficient) in order to obtain the required result in preparing solutions with the desired osmotic pressure.

There are methods of theoretical calculation of the activity coefficients, but in this treatise we have pursued a different course: we define the activity coefficient as the relation between the concentration that is calculated by means of equation II and the concentration we find by experimental determination.

2. *Available methods of determination.*

We have not made any direct determination of the osmotic pressure in an osmometer, because of the difficulty in making uniform and stable semipermeable membranes, and because it takes a longer time before an equilibrium is obtained.

It seemed natural to us, however, to consider the use of apparatus for determinations of boiling point elevations and freezing point depressions. As, however, several of the substances that are used in eye drops undergo chemical changes when boiled in aqueous solution, we abandoned the determination of the boiling point elevation. We have, on the other hand, made a large number of freezing point determinations by means of *Beckmann*'s apparatus. Actually the determination of the osmotic pressure by means of the freezing point depression can be made for all the substances that are used in the preparation of eye drops. In the case of a few substances, the solubility at 0^0 is, however, so slight that the substances can only be determined by this method in very weak concentrations, and not at all in such concentrations as are in practical use.

A determination of the vapour pressure of solutions makes it possible to work at almost the same temperature as is used when the solutions are applied practically. We had hoped to obtain dependable results by using the experimental technique employed by *Borgen (1933)*. In a dessicator were placed 12 glass beakers, 6 of which contained a sodium chloride solution of 6 %, the remaining 6 a sulphuric acid solution of 50 %. The dessicator was left closed for 24 hours at room temperature. The result was that the sulphuric acid dilutions had increased in weight, whereas the sodium chloride solutions had lost weight. The deviation, however, from the average was very great, and it was impossible to obtain reliable results, even by varying the strength of the sulphuric acid. The explanation of this is probably that the heat transfer from the dessicator to the beakers is very bad and very heterogenous. *Robinson and Sinclair (1934)* state that with a similar technique they have obtained data for the calculation of reliable activity coefficients; but these authors used silver bowls instead of glass beakers, and the bowls were placed in the dessicator on a copper plate one inch thick, so that in this way they had made sure of a good heat transfer. In later publications, however, the same authors considerably revised the values they had orginally given. So we have discarded this method of determination.

3. *Experimental technique.*

Determination of the freezing point depression by means of *Beckmann*'s thermometer is a well-known method. We have employed *Beckmann*'s macro-thermometer. For each experiment we have put 25 milliliters of solution into the container. As far as possible the supercooling has been carried each time to about 2^0 below the freezing point. At first we used a mixture of crushed ice and sodium chloride for a freezing mixture bath, but as the freezing point of the saturated solution in this case is as low as -21.2^0, it was difficult to obtain reproducible results. We found a convenient freezing mixture bath to be a mixture of crushed ice and magnesium sulphate, the freezing point of which is -3.9^0. Of course the latter bath was much slower to work with, but the results obtained were far more uniform.

According to *Ostwald-Luther* a determination of the molecular weight by means of Beckmann's macro-thermometer can be made with an accuracy of about 5 %. This requires, however, that weighings, measurements and readings are made with an accuracy of about 1 %. The chief error arises from the amount of ice disengaged in the container during the determination of the freezing point. This error can, however, easily be eliminated either by weighing the amount of disengaged ice, (which is the method we have used) or by calculation. If c is the specific heat of the solvent, λ the heat of solidification to the gramme, and v the supercooling in ^{0}C, then the fraction of the solution that freezes at the discontinuation of the supercooling is found from the following equation:

$$r = \frac{c}{\lambda} \cdot v$$

In the case of water, c = 1 and $\lambda = 79.67$. For each degree that the solution is supercooled the remaining solution is concentrated by about 1/80, or 1.25 %.

Fig. 1.

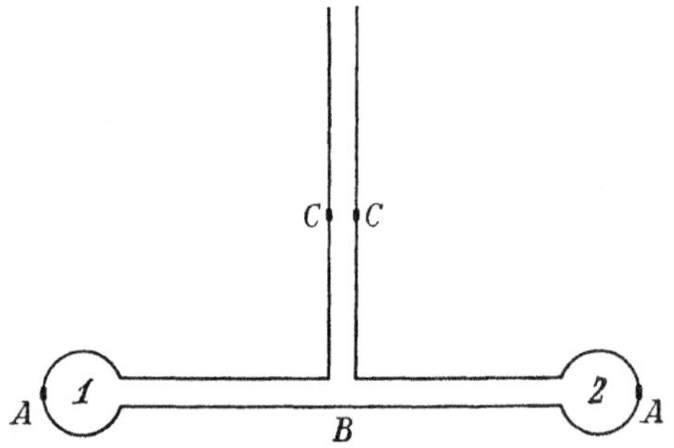

Thermocouples for measuring the vapour pressure of minute samples.
ABA: constantan wire
diameter: 0.05 mm. length: 15 mm.
AC: manganin wire
diameter: 0.05 mm.

The determination of the vapour pressure by means of *Hill's* thermoelectric method offers the great advantage that these determinations, as opposed to the freezing point determinations, are made at about 20^0. The apparatus we have used has been built in the zoophysiological laboratory at the University of Copenhagen. It was based on the principle originally stated by *Hill (1930)*, but was constructed like the modified apparatus described by *Baldes (1934)*. It consists of two thermoelements, as shown in figure 1. The way in which the various wires have been soldered together is shown at A. The two small eyes or rings (thermocouples: marked 1 and 2 in figure 1) have been insulated with a covering of a thin layer of a special varnish. A small drop of the solution, the vapour pressure of which is to be determined, is placed in one of the small rings, and a drop of the standard solution in the other. If a drop of a 0.9 % solution of sodium chloride is placed in one ring, and a drop of a 0.8 % solution of sodium chloride in the other, the difference in the rate of evaporation of the two drops will cause a difference in temperature, which will manifest itself in a thermoelectric power of 0.31×10^{-7} volts. In the galvanoscope attached to the copper-wire this power is registered, and in the apparatus we have used it showed a deflection of 50 millimetres. During the determination the part of the apparatus that is shown in the figure is kept in a brass chamber, the walls of which are lined with filter paper moistened with a solution similar to the comparison solution, which for accuracy should not differ much from the »unknown«.

It is important to pipette the solution on to the thermojunctions in a humid atmosphere, and immediately afterwards the thermocouple is placed in a moist chamber, and it is only when this chamber has been kept in the water-thermostat for about five minutes that an equilibrium is obtained, so that the determination can be made.

4. *Discussion of the errors.*

In table 1 an example is given of the original observations and the usual calculation of the equivalent concentration of NaCl, i. e. the concentration of NaCl having the same vapour pressure as a given concentration of the substance considered.

Table 1.

NaCl 8.5 ‰	$MgSO_4$ 60 ‰	M	Equivalent NaCl conc. in ‰
b → 1.6	1.5 ← a	1.55	8.73
1.2	0.8	1.00	8.65
1.3	1.5	1.40	8.71
1.3	1.1	1.20	8.68
		Mean 1.29	
NaCl 9.0 ‰	$MgSO_4$ 60 ‰	M	
1.7 ← b	a → 2.2	1.95	8.71
2.2	2.7	2.45	8.63
1.5	2.3	1.90	8.71
1.5	2.1	1.80	8.73
		Mean 2.02	8.69
		Sum 3.31	

For each two corresponding readings of the galvanometer the mean (M) is calculated. Thus, for a given concentration of NaCl we obtain a series of means, the total mean of which is computed. As the sum of the two total means corresponding to the two concentrations of NaCl is equal to the difference in galvanometer deflections which again corresponds to the difference in NaCl concentration we may calculate the equivalent NaCl concentration from each M by simple interpolation, e. g.:

$$8.50 + \frac{0.5 \cdot 1.55}{3.31} = 8.73,$$

$$9.00 - \frac{0.5 \cdot 1.95}{3.31} = 8.71.$$

The average of all such determinations is then taken as a total estimate of the concentration wanted.

The calculation may of course be somewhat simplified, in particular when the two NaCl concentrations are represented by an equal number of observations. But the figures in the last column of table 1 have been entered in order to demonstrate the uncertainty of the measurements.

The procedure is, however, open to the objection that the basis of the interpolation (3.31 in the example) has been derived from the observations themselves. Therefore, the figures in the last column of the table become correlated; thus it is not quite obvious whether the total mean is an adequate estimate of the equivalent NaCl concentration and it also seems quite obscure how we are to calculate a standard deviation that characterises the uncertainty of the measurements.

In order to overcome these difficulties we must formulate a mathematical specification of the experimental results:

In each experiment two series of galvanometer deflections are read off, one series $x_1, \ldots\ldots x_{n_1}$ against one NaCl concentration c_1, another series $y_1, \ldots\ldots y_{n_2}$ against the other NaCl concentration c_2. The x's and the y's are supposed to be normally distributed about some true values ξ and η with a common standard deviation σ, i. e.

$$x_\nu = \xi + u_\nu, \; y_\nu = \eta + v_\nu,$$

where the variances of the experimental errors are

$$\mathrm{V}\{u_\nu\} = \mathrm{V}\{v_\nu\} = \sigma^2.$$

The sum

$$\zeta = \xi + \eta$$

represents the theoretical difference in galvanometer deflection produced by the difference in NaCl concentration

$$\Delta c = c_2 - c_1.$$

The concentration of NaCl which has the same vapour pressure as the solution tested is then theoretically given by

$$\gamma = c_1 + \frac{\Delta c}{\zeta}\xi = c_2 - \frac{\Delta c}{\zeta}\eta = \frac{c_2 \xi + c_1 \eta}{\xi + \eta}.$$

Thus, putting

$$\gamma \zeta = \alpha$$

we have

$$x'_\nu = x_\nu \Delta c = \alpha - c_1 \zeta + u'_\nu$$

$$y'_\nu = y_\nu \Delta c = -\alpha + c_2 \zeta + v'_\nu$$

where the variances of

$$u'_\nu = u_\nu \Delta c \text{ and } v'_\nu = v_\nu \Delta c$$

are

$$\sigma'^2 = \sigma^2 (\Delta c)^2.$$

Now the means $\bar{x}'$ and $\bar{y}'$ render the sufficient estimates of $\alpha - c_1 \zeta$ and $-\alpha + c_2 \zeta$ and therefore

$$a = \frac{c_2 \bar{x}' + c_1 \bar{y}'}{c_2 - c_1} = c_2 \bar{x} + c_1 \bar{y}$$

and

$$z = \frac{\bar{x}' + \bar{y}'}{c_2 - c_1} = \bar{x} + \bar{y}$$

are the best possible estimates of α and ζ. The variances of a and z are

$$V\{a\} = \sigma^2 \left(\frac{c_2^2}{n_1} + \frac{c_1^2}{n_2} \right)$$

and

$$V\{z\} = \sigma^2 \left(\frac{1}{n_1} + \frac{1}{n_2} \right)$$

while the covariance is

$$V\{a, z\} = \sigma^2 \left(\frac{c_2}{n_1} + \frac{c_1}{n_2} \right)$$

As the standard errors of a and z appear to be small as compared with a and z themselves the ratio

$$c = \frac{a}{z}$$

will approximately be normally distributed about

$$\gamma = \frac{\alpha}{\zeta}$$

with a variance given by

$$\frac{V\{c\}}{\gamma^2} = \frac{V\{a\}}{\alpha^2} + \frac{V\{z\}}{\zeta^2} - 2\,\frac{V\{a,z\}}{\alpha\,\zeta}$$

or, inserting $V\{a\}$, $V\{z\}$ and $V\{a, z\}$,

$$V\{c\} = \frac{\sigma^2}{\zeta^2} \left[\frac{(c_2-\gamma)^2}{n_1} + \frac{(c_1-\gamma)^2}{n_2} \right].$$

For practical application of this formula we replace γ and ζ by c and z and σ^2 is substituted by an estimate obtained as follows: For each experimental series a sum of squares is calculated as usual:

$$SS = \sum_{\nu=1}^{n_1} (x_\nu - \bar{x})^2 + \sum_{\nu=1}^{n_2} (y_\nu - \bar{y})^2.$$

The number of degrees of freedom is $n_1 + n_2 - 2$. Next we add up the sum of squares as well as the degrees of freedom for all experimental series concerning the same substance, having first controlled, however, that the mean squares do not differ significantly from one another. For this purpose a »spurious χ^2-test« has been applied (cf. below). The pooled results have been put down in table 2.

Table 2.

Analysis of the variances of the galvanometer deflections in an experimental series.

Substance	*SS*	*f*	*MS*	„χ^2"	*P*%
Magnii sulfas	1.5126	36	0.0420	36.4	40 —50
Cincaini hydrochloridum	0.8037	14	0.0574	19.3	10 —20
Natrii bicarbonas	1.1556	18	0.0642	27.8	5 —10
Urethanum	0.3760	17	0.0221	9.0	90 —95
Kalii phosphas KH_2PO_4	0.2561	13	0.0197	6.2	90 —95
Natrii arsenas	0.7763	11	0.0706	18.7	5 —10
Pentazolum	0.1543	9	0.0171	3.7	90 —95
Antipyrinum	0.6119	17	0.0360	14.7	60 —10
Ephedrini hydrochloridum	0.8121	18	0.0451	19.5	30 —40
Kalii jodidum	1.3632	20	0.0682	32.8	2.5— 5
Natrii phosphas $Na_2HPO_4 \cdot 2H_20$	0.3320	12	0.0277	8.0	70 —80
Natrii citras	0.2984	18	0.0166	7.2	97.5—99.0
Total	8.4522	203	0.0416		

The mean squares (*MS*) certainly vary to some extent, but this is not surprising as only in one case the number of degrees of freedom (*f*) is larger than 20. Therefore it seems worth while to consider if all data might be pooled together whereby they would yield an estimated variance with numerous degrees of freedom. This variance then should be valid for all the substances. »The spurious χ^2-test« provides us with a convenient control which furthermore quite often unveils what is wrong with our hypothesis. The point in the test is: The hypothesis to be tested being that all substances under consideration have a true variance, σ^2, in common, the individual sum of squares divided by this σ^2 should vary in accordanc with the χ^2-distribution. Now the true σ^2 is of course not known, but if the hypothesis is correct the total mean square

$$s^2 = 0.0416$$

is a reliable estimate based on 203 degrees of freedom. We might therefore try, whether, when inserting 0.0416 for σ^2 we obtain a satisfactory accordance with the χ^2-distribution. For this purpose we compute the »spurious χ^2's«:

$$\frac{SS}{s^2} = {}_{\prime\prime}\chi^{2\prime\prime}$$

and consider if their distribution deviates significantly from the χ^2-distribution. In *Fisher*'s χ^2-table we read — with due regard to the degrees of freedom in each case — the probability P of a χ^2 exceeding the calculated values. These 12 P-values form the last column of table 2. Grouping them coarsely we may compare the actual distribution with the theoretical distribution:

P (%)	Number	
	found	expected
0— 10	3	1.2
10— 90	5	9.6
90—100	4	1.2
Total	12	12.0

Apparently the extreme values — i. e. large as well as small "χ^2"— are in excess. The departure from the theoretical distribution is, however, not significant and thus the test has given us no reason for rejecting the hypothesis that 0.0416 might be the true common σ^2; thus a common σ^2 may exist, and 0.0416 may be taken as an estimate of it.

If the deviation of the actual distribution from the theoretical one had been significant it might be considered whether a satisfactory agreement could be obtained by decreasing or increasing the suggested value of σ^2. The present case calls, however, for no such discussion.

As a consequence of the preceding analysis

$$s^2 = 0.0416$$

is taken as an estimate of σ^2 and

$$s = 0.204$$

as an estimate of the standard deviation σ itself.

Obviously the next step in the statistical analysis would be much simplified if the z-values could be pooled in a similar way. Considering that the standard error of z turns out to vary between 0.14 and 0.20 while the z-values in experiments with the same substance and within the same day may differ 1.0, this, however, does not seem possible. Thus, it seems advisable to determine the basis of the interpolation separately in each experimental series.

In deriving the formula for $V\{c\}$, we used an approximation, and in the practical applications it has been necessary to substitute s for σ, and the more or less accurate estimates c and z for γ and ζ. In view of these uncertainties it seems remarkable that we can solve the problem of delimiting γ exactly, and that the solution leads to a result which for practical purposes coincides with the application of the estimated standard error.

If γ is the true concentration, the quantity $a - \gamma z$ is normally distributed about 0 with the variance

$$V\{a - \gamma z\} = \sigma^2 \left(\frac{(c_2 - \gamma)^2}{n_1} + \frac{(c_1 - \gamma)^2}{n_2} \right)$$

Consequently the ratio

$$t(\gamma) = \frac{a - \gamma z}{s \sqrt{\dfrac{(c_2 - \gamma)^2}{n_1} + \dfrac{(c_1 - \gamma)^2}{n_2}}}$$

follows the t-distribution with a number of degrees of freedom equal to that used for determining s. If t_P denotes the P % limit of t, we find the P %-fiducial limits for γ by solving the inequality

$$\frac{(a - \gamma z)^2}{\dfrac{(c_2 - \gamma)^2}{n_1} + \dfrac{(c_1 - \gamma)^2}{n_2}} \leqq s^2 t_P^2$$

with regard to γ. The limits are

$$\left.\begin{matrix} \bar{c} \\ \\ \underline{c} \end{matrix}\right\} = \frac{c - \left(\dfrac{c_2}{n_1} + \dfrac{c_1}{n_2} \right) \dfrac{s^2}{z^2} t_P^2 \pm t_P \dfrac{s}{z} \sqrt{\dfrac{(c_2 - c)^2}{n_1} + \dfrac{(c_1 - c)^2}{n_2} - \dfrac{s \,\underline{\triangle}\, c}{z} \dfrac{t_P^2}{n_1 n_2}}}{1 - \left(\dfrac{1}{n_1} + \dfrac{1}{n_2} \right) \dfrac{s^2}{z^2} t_P^2}$$

where c denotes $\dfrac{a}{z}$.

The corresponding limits derived from the estimated standard error are

$$\left.\begin{array}{l}\bar{c}' \\ \underline{c}'\end{array}\right\} = c \pm t_P \frac{s}{z} \sqrt{\frac{(c_2 - c)^2}{n_1} + \frac{(c_1 - c)^2}{n_2}}$$

and they deviate from those given by the exact formula in neglecting 3 terms of the second degree in t_p. The difference is, however, of no consequence as 1) the supplementary term under the square root amounts to at most 1‰ of the main term; 2) the total correction effected by the two other supplementary terms has a mean value which is only about $^1/_3$ of the mean error.

This analysis shows that there is every good reason for applying the simpler procedure for calculating the estimated standard error.

Table 3.

Calculation of the estimate of the equivalent NaCl concentration c and its standard error $SE\{c\}$.

Substance Concentration	c_1	c_2	n_1	n_2	$\bar{x}$	$\bar{y}$	a	z	c	$10^4 \cdot V\{c\}$	$10^2 \cdot SE\{c\}$
Magnii sulfas											
60 ‰	8.5	9.0	4	4	1.2875	2.0250	28.800	3.3125	8.694	1.24	1.11
»	8.5	9.0	4	4	0.8625	2.2250	26.675	3.0875	8.640	1.63	1.28
»	8.5	9.0	4	4	0.9750	1.8500	24.500	2.8250	8.673	1.78	1.33
»	8.5	9.0	4	4	0.6000	2.2000	24.100	2.8000	8.607	2.20	1.48
»	8.5	9.0	4	4	0.8375	2.2250	26.450	3.0625	8.637	1.67	1.29
»	8.5	9.0	4	4	0.8125	2.1500	25.588	2.9625	8.637	1.78	1.33
Cincaini hydrochloridum											
60 ‰	4.0	4.5	2	3	0.3250	2.2667	10.529	2.5917	4.063	6.00	2.45
45 ‰	3.5	4.0	2	2	1.5750	1.0000	9.800	2.5750	3.806	4.12	2.03
30 ‰	3.0	3.5	3	3	1.0000	1.4500	7.850	7.4500	3.204	2.99	1.73
15 ‰	1.5	2.0	2	3	1.5250	1.1167	4.725	2.6417	1.789	3.02	1.74
Natrii bicarbonas											
20 ‰	12.5	13.0	4	4	1.1625	1.2125	30.269	2.3750	12.745	2.31	1.52
15 ‰	9.5	10.0	3	3	1.2667	1.5333	27.233	2.8000	9.726	2.24	1.50
10 ‰	6.0	6.5	3	2	2.2167	0.4500	17.109	2.6667	6.416	5.21	2.28
5 ‰	3.0	3.5	3	4	1.3833	1.4000	9.042	2.7833	3.249	1.96	1.40
Urethanum											
40 ‰	12.0	12.5	3	3	0.8667	1.8667	33.234	2.7334	12.159	2.63	1.62
20 ‰	5.5	6.0	3	4	2.0667	0.7750	16.663	2.8417	5.864	2.03	1.42
9.7 ‰	2.5	3.0	3	3	0.8500	1.4667	6.217	2.3167	2.684	3.46	1.86
5 ‰	1.0	1.5	3	3	1.1667	1.2500	3.000	2.4167	1.241	2.98	1.73
Kalii phosphas KH_2PO_4											
30 ‰	12.0	12.5	3	2	0.7333	2.2250	35.866	2.9583	12.124	2.61	1.62
20 ‰	8.0	8.5	3	3	1.5833	1.0667	21.992	2.6500	8.299	2.56	1.60
15 ‰	6.0	6.5	2	2	1.6000	0.8750	15.650	2.4750	6.323	4.61	2.15
7.5 ‰	3.0	3.5	3	3	0.9667	1.0833	6.633	2.0500	3.236	4.14	2.03

Table continued on next page

Substance Concentration	c_1	c_2	n_1	n_2	$\bar{x}$	$\bar{y}$	a	z	c	$10^4 \cdot V\{c\}$	$10^2 \cdot SE\{c\}$
Natrii arsenas											
40 ‰	9.0	9.5	3	3	1.7500	0.7000	22.925	2.4500	9.357	3.42	1.85
20 ‰	4.5	5.0	2	3	1.3000	1.2000	11.900	2.5000	4.760	3.42	1.85
10 ‰	2.0	2.5	2	2	1.7250	1.2000	6.712	2.9250	2.295	3.13	1.77
5 ‰	1.0	1.5	2	2	1.2500	1.2000	3.075	2.4500	1.255	4.34	2.08
Pentazolum											
60 ‰	10.5	11.0	2	3	1.5000	1.0833	27.875	2.5833	10.790	3.12	1.77
30 ‰	6.0	6.5	2	2	1.7500	0.6250	15.125	2.3750	6.368	5.64	2.37
15 ‰	3.0	3.5	2	2	0.7750	1.7500	7.962	2.5250	3.153	4.69	2.17
Antipyrinum											
60 ‰	8.0	8.5	2	3	1.3000	1.2167	20.784	2.5167	8.258	3.38	1.84
45 ‰	6.0	6.5	3	3	1.8000	0.7333	16.100	2.5333	6.355	3.18	1.78
30 ‰	4.0	4.5	3	3	1.8333	1.0167	12.317	2.8500	4.322	2.32	1.52
7.5 ‰	1.0	1.5	3	3	0.5667	1.8667	2.717	2.4334	1.117	3.76	1.94
Ephedrini hydrochloridum											
50 ‰	14.0	14.5	4	2	0.6500	1.9000	36.025	2.5500	14.127	2.74	1.66
25 ‰	6.5	7.0	3	3	2.4333	0.2667	18.767	2.7000	6.951	3.92	1.98
12.5 ‰	3.0	3.5	3	5	2.7000	0.3100	10.380	3.0100	3.449	1.89	1.37
6.25 ‰	1.5	2.0	3	3	1.6833	0.6500	4.342	2.3333	1.861	3.82	1.95
Kalii jodidum											
20 ‰	6.5	7.0	4	4	2.4500	0.3625	19.506	2.8125	6.935	2.54	1.59
10 ‰	3.0	3.5	4	4	2.0000	1.0875	10.262	3.0875	3.324	1.49	1.22
5 ‰	1.5	2.0	4	3	1.1250	1.8000	4.950	2.9250	1.692	1.75	1.32
Natrii phosphas $Na_2HPO_4 2H_2O$											
30 ‰	12.0	12.5	3	2	0.2000	2.8750	37.000	3.0750	12.033	3.22	1.79
20 ‰	8.0	8.5	3	2	0.8333	1.7250	20.883	2.5583	8.163	3.25	1.80
15 ‰	6.0	6.5	3	2	0.5500	1.9000	14.975	2.4500	6.112	3.91	1.98
7.5 ‰	3.0	3.5	3	2	0.6667	1.9750	8.258	2.6417	3.126	3.25	1.80
Natrii citras											
50 ‰	14.0	14.5	2	3	2.4000	0.3167	39.234	2.7167	14.442	3.77	1.94
40 ‰	11.5	12.0	2	3	1.7750	1.0833	33.758	2.8583	11.811	2.55	1.60

Table 3 gives a synopsis of the calculations concerning the experiments with various concentrations of several substances. From the last column we may read that *on the whole the uncertainty of the determination of the equivalent concentration of NaCl is characterised by a standard error of 0.0011—0.0025, the exact value depending on the design and the results of each experimental series.*

As to the true value of the concentration γ, it is usually (i. e. in 95 % of the cases) expected to lie within a margin of between $\pm$ 0.0022 and $\pm$ 0.0050 about the c value observed.

In the above only the experimental error under optimal conditions has been discussed, the determinations considered having been made in direct succession. If several series of experiments are made during a single day, amongst other things, the temperature of the room will vary, and we find that the results deviate more than was to be expected from the standard error determined above. Table 3 e. g. shows that the c values found for $MgSO_4$ vary between

Table 4.

Calculations for repeated determinations of equivalent NaCl concentrations.

Substance	Conc. in ‰	c_1	c_2	n_1	n_2	$\bar{x}$	$\bar{y}$	a	z	k	$10^4 \cdot V\{c\}$	$10^2 \cdot SE\{c\}$
Procaini hydrochloridum												
15 VII 42	15.0	2.5	3.0	3	3	1.4167	0.8000	0.6250	2.2167	0.2820	3.81	1.95
16 VII 42	15.0	2.5	3.0	2	2	1.6500	0.5500	0.6325	2.2000	0.2875	6.72	2.59
Aneurini hydrochloridum												
22 VIII 42	30.0	6.0	6.5	2	3	2.8000	0.1833	1.9300	7.9833	0.6469	3.45	1.86
30 IX 42	30.0	6.0	6.5	4	5	1.5750	1.4100	1.8698	2.9850	0.6264	1.30	1.14
Tropacocaini hydrochloridum												
21 II 46	50.0	9.0	9.5	3	2	0.6167	2.1000	2.4759	2.7167	0.9114	3.17	1.78
2 IV 46	50.0	9.0	9.5	3	2	0.8500	1.9500	2.5625	2.8000	0.9152	2.72	1.65
Optochini hydrochloridum												
25 III 45	50.0	4.5	5.0	3	2	0.8667	2.6750	1.6371	3.5417	0.4622	1.83	1.35
29 IX 45	50.0	4.0	4.5	3	3	1.0667	2.0333	1.2933	3.1000	0.4172	1.98	1.41
Codeini phosphas												
8 X 42	7.5	0.5	1.0	2	3	2.1000	0.5667	0.2383	2.6667	0.0894	3.36	1.83
28 VIII 43	7.5	0.5	1.0	3	3	2.3500	0.4833	0.2592	2.8333	0.0915	3.10	1.76

8.607 and 8.694, which is 4.7 times the standard error of their difference. It is true, this evalution is not correct, as the values considered are extreme, but if a weighted mean square is calculated for all 6 values, we get 0.246, which divided by the variance s^2 = 0.0416, gives a variance ratio $v^2 = 5.92$, and from *Fisher*'s Table we see that this value differs significantly from 1 ($P < 0.1$ %). This implies that the equivalent concentration of NaCl does not constantly take values within the experimental error determined.

The above to a still greater degree applies to substances that have been tested twice at intervals of some time. Table 4 gives the complete calculations for 5 duplicate determinations, and in Table 5 the differences between corresponding determinations have been entered. Two of the differences are very large compared with the calculated standard error.

Table 5.
Comparison between repeated vapour pressure determinations.

Substance	Concentration in ‰	Dates	d	$10^4 \cdot V\{d\}$	$SE\{d\}$	t
Procaini hydrochloridum	15.0	15 VII 41—16 VII 42	0.055	10.53	0.032	1.7
Aneurini hydrochloridum	30.0	22 VIII 42—30 IX 42	0.205	4.75	0.022	9.3
Tropacocaini hydrochloridum	50.0	21 II 46—2 IV 46	0.038	5.89	0.024	1.6
Optochini hydrochloridum	50.0	25 III 45—29 IX 45	0.450	3.81	0.020	22.5
Codeini phosphas	7.5	8 X 42—28 VIII 43	0.021	6.46	0.025	0.8

In reality, this fact is not very astonishing. When two determinations are made in direct succession, the sources of error which lead to the total experimental error will to a large degree be the same in both cases, and their contribution to the total error will therefore be repeated. During a day some of the sources of error, e. g. the temperature of the room, will vary, and if the determinations are made at longer intervals, still more factors will be of effect: new dilutions may have been made, the insulating coating of varnish on the thermocouple may have been renewed, the galvanometer have been repaired, etc., etc. — all of which are things which must actually be considered as contributing to the total experimental error when, as in the present case, the aim is to determine a curve of freezing points at one time and in one place and which can be used in other laboratories for standardisation of solutions to be used there.

A direct determination of the variation of the total experimental error would demand, that during the whole period during which experiments have been made, different dilutions of e. g. $MgSO_4$ had constantly been controlled against fresh solutions of both $MgSO_4$ and NaCl. As such experiments have not been made, a direct discussion of the errors is not possible.

Table 6.
14 control experiments on the standardisation of solutions to the point of isotonicity with about 9 ‰ NaCl.

Substance	In 100 grm. solution: Amount (grm.)	In 100 grm. solution: added NaCl (grm.)	Freezing point depression (°C): Substance	Freezing point depression (°C): NaCl	Mixture	Equivalent NaCl Concentration (‰): Calculated	Equivalent NaCl Concentration (‰): Determined	Equivalent NaCl Concentration (‰): Difference
Scopolamini hydrobromidum	0.10	0.90	0.005	0.520	0.525	9.05	8.95	+ 0.10
Atropini sulfas	0.20	0.90	0.015	0.520	0.535	9.25	9.05	+ 0.20
Atropini sulfas	0.50	0.85	0.040	0.500	0.540	9.35	9.00	+ 0.35
Homatropini hydrobromidum	0.50	0.85	0.049	0.500	0.549	9.50	9.05	+ 0.45
Zinci sulfas	0.30	0.80	0.030	0.465	0.495	8.60	8.40	+ 0.20
Zinci sulfas	0.30	0.85	0.030	0.495	0.525	9.05	8.85	+ 0.20
Physostigmini salicylas	1.00	0.75	0.090	0.435	0.525	9.05	8.85	+ 0.20
Aneurini hydrochloridum	1.00	0.70	0.140	0.405	0.545	9.45	9.10	+ 0.35
Cocaini hydrochloridum	2.00	0.65	0.175	0.380	0.555	9.60	9.20	+ 0.40
Cocaini hydrochloridum	2.00	0.60	0.175	0.350	0.525	9.05	9.00	+ 0.05
Aethylmorphini hydrochloridum	2.00	0.65	0.174	0.380	0.554	9.60	9.00	+ 0.60
Pilocarpini hydrochloridum	2.00	0.50	0.255	0.295	0.540	9.35	9.20	+ 0.15
Emetini hydrochloridum	5.00	0.40	0.275	0.240	0.515	8.90	8.40	+ 0.50
Emetini hydrochloridum	5.00	0.45	0.275	0.265	0.540	9.35	8.95	+ 0.40

From some of the data we can, however, evaluate how the practical results with the technique for standardising a solution of some substance together with NaCl to the point of isotonicity with 9 ‰ NaCl, based on the freezing point depression curves, present themselves.

The procedure is as follows: If e. g. we wish to make a 5.0 ‰ solution of atropin, we read from the curve that this concentration causes a freezing point depression of 0.040°; in order to obtain the depression of 0.520° corresponding to 9.0 ‰ NaCl, the solution is made 8.5 ‰ in NaCl, which corresponds to a depression of 0.500°. If we assumed, that the depression of the mixture is 0.040° + 0.500° = 0.540°, it would be isotonic with 9.35 ‰ NaCl; experimental control gives the value 9.00 ‰. 14 such controls for different solutions have been put down in table 6, the last column of which gives the differences between the calculated and the experimentally determined concentration of NaCl which are equivalent to the mixtures.

All these differences are positive, so that first of all we may state *that the method has a systematic error, which for the cases considered here averages 0.30 ‰ NaCl.*

Besides this we have the random variations, the standard deviation of which is estimated at 0.162 ‰; in practical work this means: *When a calculated equivalent concentration of NaCl near 9 ‰ has been corrected for the systematic error, a further margin of uncertainty has to be considered, namely* $\pm$ *2.16 · 0.162 ‰ =* $\pm$ *0.35 ‰*. The factor 2.16 is the 95 % limit in »Student's« t-distribution with 13 degrees of freedom.

As in chemical determinations the uncertainty margin is generally given in percentage, we may state that the estimate of the standard deviation is found to be 1.8 % and the uncertainty margin ± 3.9 % out of the about 9 ‰ NaCl aimed at. It must, however, be pointed out that in the present work no data are available for determining the uncertainty at other concentration levels of NaCl.

III. THE PREPARATION OF ISOOSMOTIC EYE DROPS

1. Previous investigations concerning the composition of lachrymal fluid, and the requirements that ideal eye drops should fulfil.

Eye drops were first introduced into *Pharmacopoea Helvetica 1933* and into *Dispensatorium Danicum 1934*. In making these solutions the end in view was to obtain isoosmosis with the lachrymal fluid on the supposition that the latter had the same osmotic pressure as a sodium chloride solution of 1.4 %.

We have been informed *(by Professor Eder of Zürich)* that all the values stated in *Ph. Helv.* originate from a work by *Lumière & Chevrotier (1913)*. These values were not checked up prior to publication in *Ph. Helv.*, from which they have since been indiscriminately reprinted in various textbooks, for instance *Remington's Practice of Pharmacy*. *Lumière & Chevrotier* gained great credit by making an appeal for the use of isotonic solutions, not only for parenteral injections, but also for use in the treatment of mucous membranes, where nasal, laryngeal, vaginal, vesical, urethral, or eye irrigations are involved. They gave values for use in the calculation of the various concentrations of active substances and auxiliary substances. The values were based on a number of freezing point determinations. No details concerning the technique used in these determinations were given. It was stated that no special, chemically pure substances had been used, but only commercial samples. It was taken for granted that the freezing point of blood serum was 0.56°, and that of lachrymal fluid was 0.80°. Moreover, *Lumière & Chevrotier* were of opinion that the most important thing was to avoid hypotonic solutions, and therefore proposed that eye drops in many cases could be prepared simply by dissolving the active substance in a 1.4 % solution of sodium chloride. In the debate which has been going on about the correct composition of eye drops, the most important consideration has, no doubt, been the desire to be able to make such solutions as do not cause pain when applied (fortiter in re, suaviter in modo), and here the interest has, in the main, been focussed on the question of osmosis.

By means of the *hæmolytic* method for determining the reciprocal osmotic condition of solutions (introduced by *Hamburger* in 1883), the statement was arrived at that a 0.9 % solution of sodium chloride was isoosmotic with blood. When *Massart (1889) and Hamburger (1906)* by their examinations of the lachrymal fluid found that it should correspond with a 1.4 % solution of sodium chloride, that statement has, till now, passed uncontradicted. *Oguchi (1922)* also quotes *Hamburger*, but at the same time adds that *Sudo* should have found the value to be 1 %. *Oguchi* has not himself analysed the composition of the lachrymal fluid, but by instilling solutions of sodium chloride of different concentrations into the eye, he has found that solutions between 1.0 and 1.4 % do not cause the sensation of pain that is prevalent at the instillation of solutions of 0.5 and 2.0 %. Indirect tests like this one are faulty because of the subjective factors that make themselves felt. Actually *Hamburger*'s direct determinations were accurate, but, as will be understood, the greatest difficulty lies in the collection of the lachrymal fluid to be analysed. Examinations made by *Krogh, Lund, and Pedersen-Bjergaard (1945)* show that the lachrymal fluid has the same osmotic pressure as blood, corresponding to a 0.9 % solution of sodium chloride. The same value is stated in *Lundsgaard*'s »Lærebog i Fysiologi«.

As to the correct concentration of eye drops (with reference to osmosis), it must be realized that other considerations may be indicated than complete absence of pain. Thus *Oguchi* maintains that a very quick and thorough effect is obtained by applying anosmotic solutions, because in this way the epithelium of the cornea is strained. This effect, however, is rather transitory, because this straining of the epithelium causes a pain, followed by a greatly increased secretion of tears, which weakens the effect because of dilution. In keeping with this, *Bossalino* (1938) finds that the absorption of pilocarpine is slowest from isoosmotic solutions, and more rapid from both hyper- and hypotonic solutions.

The sensation of pain caused by the application of eye drops is, however, also caused by other factors than the conditions of osmotic concentration. *Oguchi* has called attention to the fact that the solutions must not be too cold when instilled into the eye. Furthermore the acidity of the solution is of the greatest importance. This was shown by *Oguchi & Nakashima (1927)*. These two authors were of opinion that the pH of the lachrymal fluid was between 8.4 and 8.6, but that eye drops of pH 7.8 caused least pain. *Roulet (1923)* also found that pH 7.8 was best suited for the purpose. *Hosford & Hicks (1935)* quote both the examinations of these, and of other authors. After a critical review of the methods employed for the determinations, *Hosford & Hicks* find that the lachrymal fluid has the same pH as blood: 7.35. Referring to a report from *Dr. W. Hess* of Zürich, the same result is stated by *Büchi & Baeschlin (1936)*.

To complete the picture it is mentioned that the oxidation-reduction potential may be of great importance to the sensation of pain e. g. in the case of solutions of methylene blue *(Henrioul 1936)*.

2. Own investigations.

In the present work we have determined the freezing point depression or the vapour pressure, and sometimes we have made both the determinations, of aqueous solutions of the substances that are usually contained in eye drops. When we started the work, we assumed that eye drops were to be adjusted to a freezing point depression of 0.80°, corresponding to a sodium chloride solution of 1.4 %, and we had almost concluded the determinations, when *Krogh, Lund & Pedersen-Bjergaard (1945)* in determinations of lachrymal fluid from 10 individuals pointed out that the lachrymal fluid, like blood, corresponds to a sodium chloride solution of 0.9 %. As, however, there is a possibility of occasional applications of hyperosmotic solutions, as mentioned above, we have, after all, included all the results of our determinations in the present treatise, that is also the results between the freezing point depression of 0.52° and 0.80°, which represent the hyperosmotic solutions.

3. Substances examined.

In this examination we have included all the substances found among the eye drops of the Dispensatorium Danicum, and also some other substances that are generally used in extemporaneous prescriptions of eye drops.

To find out which concentration of the substances would be most suitable for the determinations, we made a number of calculations, the results of which are given in table 7. The calculation have been made by inserting the respective values in equation II.

Table 7.
A list of the 28 substances included in the present examination.

							A graphical representation of		
							I The values calculated according to Raoult's law	II A comparison between the calculated and the experimentally found values	III The values found experimentally and for practical use shown together with the mirrored NaCl curve
n		M.	0.20°	0.40°	0.56°	0.80°	found in figure		
1	Acidum boricum	61.84	0.665	1.330	1.862	2.660	3	7	12
2	Adrenalini bitartras	333.16	1.791	3.582	5.015	7.164	2	9	14
2	Adrenoni hydrochloridum	217.57	1.170	2.340	3.275	4.680	2	11	14
2	Aethylmorphini hydrochloridum	385.69	2.073	4.147	5.806	8.294	3	10	15
3	Aluminii kalii sulfas	474.38	1.700	3.400	4.761	6.801	3	11	15
2	Alypini hydrochloridum	314.69	1.698	3.384	4.737	6.767	2	8	13
2	Argenti nitras	169.89	0.913	1.827	2.557	3.654	2	10	16
	Argyrolum							10	16
2	Atropini sulfas	694.48	3.734	7.468	10.455	14.935	2	7	12
2	Cocaini hydrochloridum	339.65	1.826	3.652	5.113	7.304	3	7	12
2	Cupri sulfas	279.71	1.343	2.685	3.759	5.370	2	7	14
2	Ephedrini hydrochloridum	201.60	1.084	2.168	3.035	4.335	3	8	12
3	Fluoresceinnatrium	376.08	1.348	2.695	3.775	5.390	3	11	14
2	Homatropini hydrobromidum	356.11	1.914	3.829	5.369	7.658	2	11	12
2	Kalii chloras	122.56	0.659	1.318	1.846	2.636	2	8	15
2	Kalii nitras	101.11	0.544	1.087	1.522	2.174	3	9	16
2	Methylatropini nitras	366.23	1.970	3.940	5.515	7.880	3	9	13
3	Natrii boras	381.44	1.367	2.734	3.828	5.469	2	9	12
2	Natrii chloridum	58.46	0.314	0.629	0.880	1.254	2	5—6	12—15
2	Optochini hydrochloridum	376.71	2.025	4.050	5.671	8.100	2	11	13
2	Phenacainæ hydrochloridum	334.66	1.799	3.598	5.037	7.196	3	8	13
2	Physostigmini salicylas	413.25	2.222	4.443	6.220	8.886	2	9	14
2	Pilocarpini hydrochloridum	244.62	1.315	2.630	3.682	5.261	2	7	12
1	Resorcinum	110.05	1.183	2.367	3.314	4.733	3	10	15
2	Scopolamini hydrobromidum	438.15	2.356	4.711	6.596	9.422	3	8	14
	Targesinum							10	16
2	Tropacocaini hydrochloridum	245.16	1.318	2.636	3.692	5.272	3	10	13
2	Zinci sulfas	287.55	1.546	3.092	4.329	6.184	3	7	12

Against each substance, we have, where it has been possible, given the number of ions, into which the substance is supposed to be dissociated, the molecular weight and the percentages of the concentration that should be supposed to give a freezing point depression of 0.20°, 0.40°, 0.56° and 0.80° respectively, calculated by equation II.

The values stated in table 7 are given graphically in figures 2 and 3.

Fig. 2

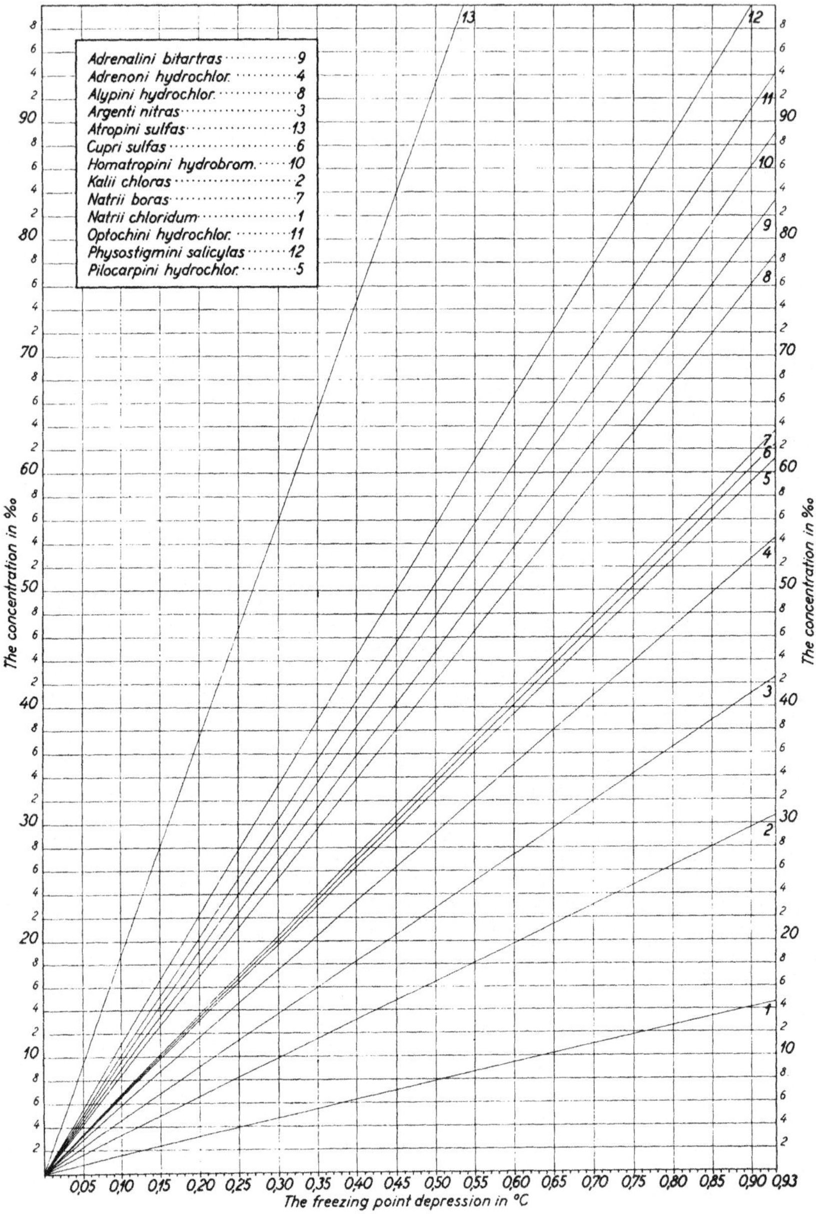

Adrenalini bitartras ··· 9
Adrenoni hydrochlor. ··· 4
Alypini hydrochlor. ··· 8
Argenti nitras ··· 3
Atropini sulfas ··· 13
Cupri sulfas ··· 6
Homatropini hydrobrom. ··· 10
Kalii chloras ··· 2
Natrii boras ··· 7
Natrii chloridum ··· 1
Optochini hydrochlor. ··· 11
Physostigmini salicylas ··· 12
Pilocarpini hydrochlor. ··· 5
The concentration in ‰
The freezing point depression in °C
0,05 0,10 0,15 0,20 0,25 0,30 0,35 0,40 0,45 0,50 0,55 0,60 0,65 0,70 0,75 0,80 0,85 0,90 0,93
10 20 30 40 50 60 70 80 90

Fig. 3

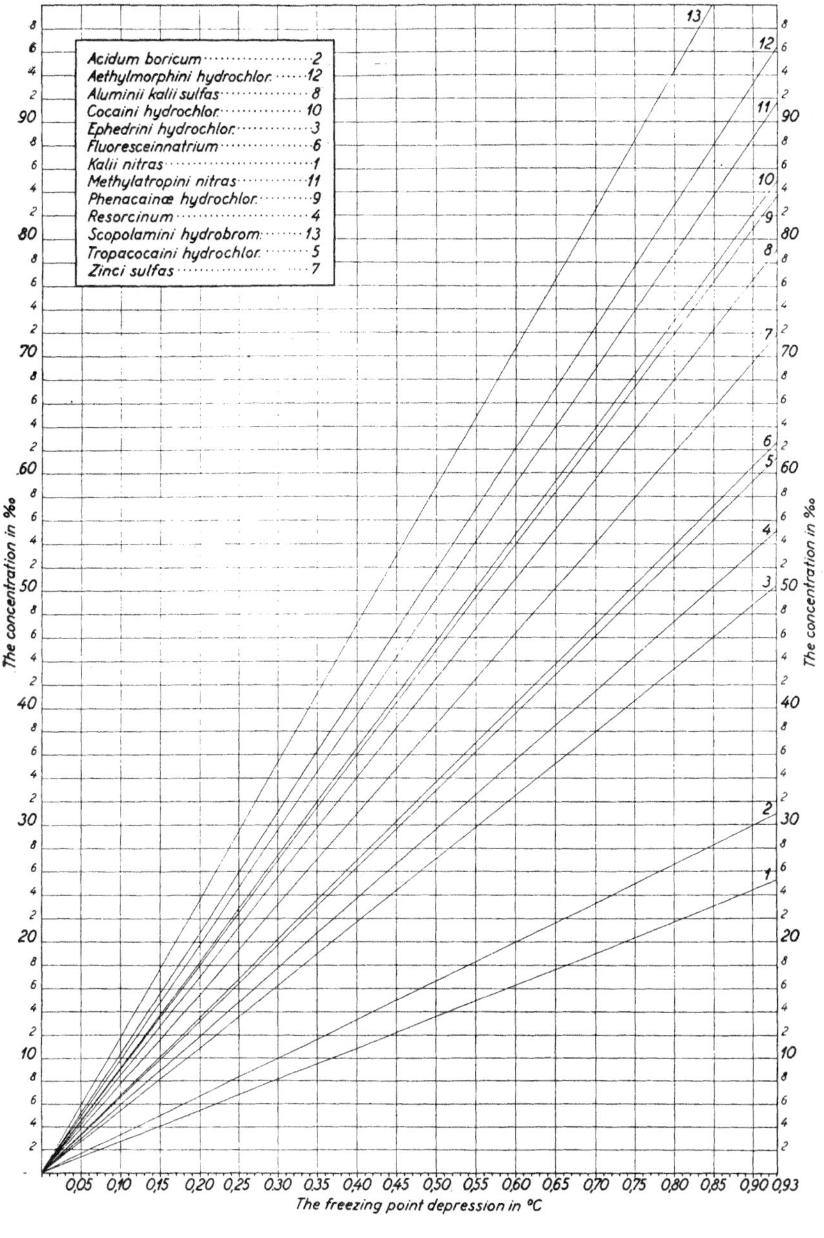

Acidum boricum 2
Aethylmorphini hydrochlor. 12
Aluminii kalii sulfas 8
Cocaini hydrochlor. 10
Ephedrini hydrochlor. 3
Fluoresceinnatrium 6
Kalii nitras 1
Methylatropini nitras 11
Phenacainæ hydrochlor. 9
Resorcinum 4
Scopolamini hydrobrom. 13
Tropacocaini hydrochlor. 5
Zinci sulfas 7
The concentration in ‰
The freezing point depression in °C
0,05 0,10 0,15 0,20 0,25 0,30 0,35 0,40 0,45 0,50 0,55 0,60 0,65 0,70 0,75 0,80 0,85 0,90 0,93
10 20 30 40 50 60 70 80 90

In figures 2 and 3 the concentration of the substances is marked in ⁰/₀₀ (per thousand) along the ordinate. The freezing point depression is marked in °C along the abscissa. The curves that show the steepest course represent substances with high molecular weights, whereas the curves showing the flattest course represent substances with low molecular weights. At the same time substances that are only slightly dissociated show a curve with a steeper course than more dissociated substances with molecule weights of the same magnitude.

Although the values given in figures 2 and 3 are calculated theoretically, we should like to show by an example how the figures obtained might be used practically. Assuming the freezing point depression of a 0.9 % solution of sodium chloride not to be 0.56° as calculated and stated in table 7, but 0.52°, (which result we have reached by means of our determinations, as will be accounted for later on in this treatise). If, for instance, a solution containing 1 % of resorcinol is to be prepared in such a way that it becomes iso-

Fig. 4

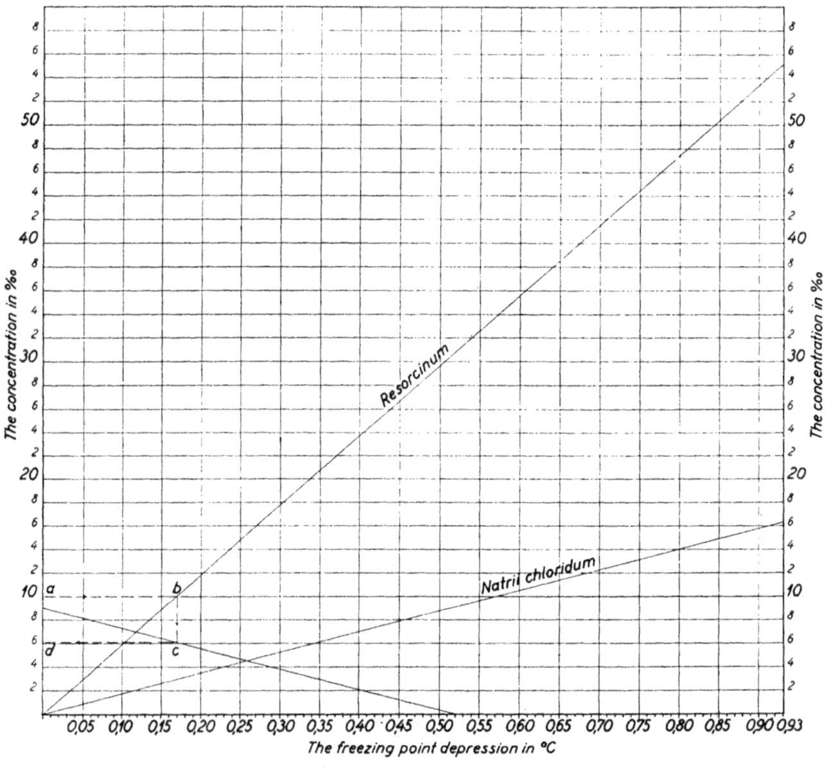

osmotic with the lachrymal fluid, by adding to it the necessary amount of sodium chloride, it is seen from fig. 4 that a 1 % solution of resorcinol gives an osmotic pressure corresponding to a freezing point depression of 0.17^{0}. The amount of sodium chloride which is then to be added must give a freezing point depression of $0.52^{0} - 0.17^{0} = 0.35^{0}$, which in fig. 4 is seen to correspond with a 0.61 % solution of sodium chloride. That is to say that a solution of 100 grammes, containing 1 gramme of resorcinol and 61 centigrammes of sodium chloride, will be isoosmotic with the lachrymal fluid, or a 0.9 % solution of sodium chloride. By drawing a »mirrored« sodium chloride curve, starting from the point on the abscissa that corresponds to the freezing point depression at which the prepared solution is to be fixed, it is possible to read directly the difference resulting from the above calculation (0.35^{0}), as will be seen from the dotted line in fig. 4 (a—b—c—d).

4. The double logarithmic system of coordinates.

If a function is required to be shown graphically, for instance $v = a \cdot u$, this is generally done by marking u and v along the abscissa and the ordinate in a linear system of coordinates.

A double logarithmic system is the result, however, if the values of u and v are not marked directly, but instead $x = \log u$ and $y = \log v$.

A straight line in the logarithmic system can be written in the following form

$$y = a \cdot x + b$$

or

$$\log v = a \cdot \log u + b$$

The antilogarithm of this equation is

$$v = u^{a} \cdot 10^{b}$$

or, as 10^{b} is a constant (c),

$$v = c \cdot u^{a}$$

This is the expression of the corresponding curve in the arithmetical system. It will be seen that a is the inclination of the straight line in the logarithmic system. If $a = 1$ the straight line will have such a course as to cut the ordinate at an angle of 45^{0}, if the abscissa and the ordinate are divided in the same way as in fig. 5. This is, for instance the case with all the calculated relations between the concentration and the freezing point depression, which relations also give straight lines in the arithmetical system. If a is greater than 1, the straight line in the logarithmic system has a more perpendicular course, and the angle it forms with the ordinate becomes smaller than 45°, that is to say, the corresponding curve in the arithmetical system becomes a parabolic shape, the axis of which is the ordinate. If a is smaller than 1, the straight line in the logarithmic system has a more horizontal course, and the angle becomes greater than 45°, which means that the curve in the arithmetical system forms a parabolic figure the axis of which is the abscissa.

On the basis of the determined sodium chloride values the following pages will give an instance of the calculation of the relations between the concentration and the freezing point depression in the arithmetical system.

Natrii chloridum.

Freezing point determinations were made of the following solutions of sodium chloride. At each determination the amount of disengaged ice was weighed, and the concentration of sodium chloride corrected accordingly. The result is seen in table 8.

Table 8.

The concentration in ‰	14.0	14.0	14.0	14.0	14.0	13.3	13.3	12.6	10.0	9.0	5.0	2.3
The corrected concentration in ‰	14.7	14.7	14.7	14.7	14.7	14.0	14.0	13.3	10.7	9.7	5.5	2.5
The freezing point depression in °C.	0.845	0.847	0.850	0.848	0.850	0.801	0.797	0.750	0.616	0.560	0.320	0.150

The straight line drawn in fig. 5, symbolising sodium chloride, is synonymous with the following mathematical expression for the relationship found between the freezing point depression and the concentration:

As the relationship between the concentration and the freezing point depression is indicated by means of a straight line, this interdependence must, according to the above, find its expression in the following formula:

$$K = c \cdot F^{a}$$

in which K is the concentration, and F the freezing point depression.

The constants a and c must be determined from the knowledge of 2 points (F_1, K_1) and (F_2, K_2). We then have:

$$K_1 = c \cdot F_1^a$$

$$K_2 = c \cdot F_2^a$$

$$\frac{K_1}{K_2} = \frac{F_1^a}{F_2^a}$$

$$K_1 \cdot F_2^a = K_2 \cdot F_1^a$$

$$\log K_1 + a \cdot \log F_2 = \log K_2 + a \cdot \log F_1$$

$$a = \frac{\log K_1 - \log K_2}{\log F_1 - \log F_2}$$

When thus a has been found, c can be determined from the equation:

$$K_1 = c \cdot F_1^a$$

If two pairs of experimental values of sodium chloride, $(F_1, K_1) = (0.52; 9)$ and $(F_2, K_2) = (0.15; 2.5)$, are inserted into this equation, the equation of sodium chloride in the arithmetical system is found to be:

$$K = 17.65 \cdot F^{1.03}$$

K being the concentration expressed in ‰ and F the freezing point depression in °C.

In table 9 it is seen how the calculations have been made, to make it possible to draw the straight line in figure 5 in the logarithmic system. In cases where more than one determination have been made of the same concentration, the average has been calculated.

Table 9.

The concentration in ‰	log concentration	The freezing point depression	log freezing point depression
14.7	1.1673	0.848	0.9284 — 1 = — 0.0716
14.0	1.1461	0.799	0.9025 — 1 = — 0.0975
13.3	1.1239	0.750	0.8751 — 1 = — 0.1249
10.7	1.0294	0.616	0.7896 — 1 = — 0.2104
9.7	0.9868	0.560	0.7482 — 1 = — 0.2518
5.5	0.7404	0.320	0.5051 — 1 = — 0.4949
2.5	0.3979	0.150	0.1761 — 1 = — 0.8232

In table 10 there are a number of calculations of the freezing point depressions of sodium chloride solutions of given concentrations, calculated by means of the equation:

$$K = 17.65 \cdot F^{1.03}$$

and these figures have been used at the drawing of the curve in the arithmetical system in fig. 6. All our determinations with *Hill's* apparatus were based on this sodium chloride curve: when by means of the vapour pressure determination we found the sodium chloride solution that corresponded to a given solution of a given substance, the result was converted into a freezing point depression by means of the curve.

Table 10.
K: the concentration of NaCl in ‰.
F: the freezing point depression in °C.

K	F	K	F	K	F	K	F
0.0	0.000	5.0	0.294	10.0	0.576	15.0	0.854
0.5	0.031	5.5	0.322	10.5	0.604	15.5	0.882
1.0	0.062	6.0	0.351	11.0	0.632	16.0	0.909
1.5	0.091	6.5	0.379	11.5	0.660	16.5	0.937
2.0	0.121	7.0	0.407	12.0	0.688	17.0	0.964
2.5	0.150	7.5	0.436	12.5	0.715	17.5	0.992
3.0	0.179	8.0	0.464	13.0	0.743		
3.5	0.208	8.5	0.492	13.5	0.771		
4.0	0.237	9.0	0.520	14.0	0.799		
4.5	0.265	9.5	0.548	14.5	0.826		

Using the logarithmic system of coordinates we have the advantage that on the basis of a few observations the straight line can be drawn that denotes the relation between the freezing point depression and the concentration, whereas the more or less arched curve, which is the result in the arithmetical system, will demand many more observations if it is to be drawn fairly accurately. An example of the logarithmic system is seen in fig. 5. The logarithm of the freezing point depression, expressed in °C, has been marked along the abscissa, and the logarithm of the concentration, expressed in ‰, along the ordinate. The calculated straight line for sodium chloride is dotted, while the experimental straight line has been drawn through the greatest possible number of determined values. The vertical line gives the freezing point depression of 0.52°, the point of intersection of this vertical line and the straight line for sodium chloride gives the isoosmotic concentration of this substance.

Fig. 5

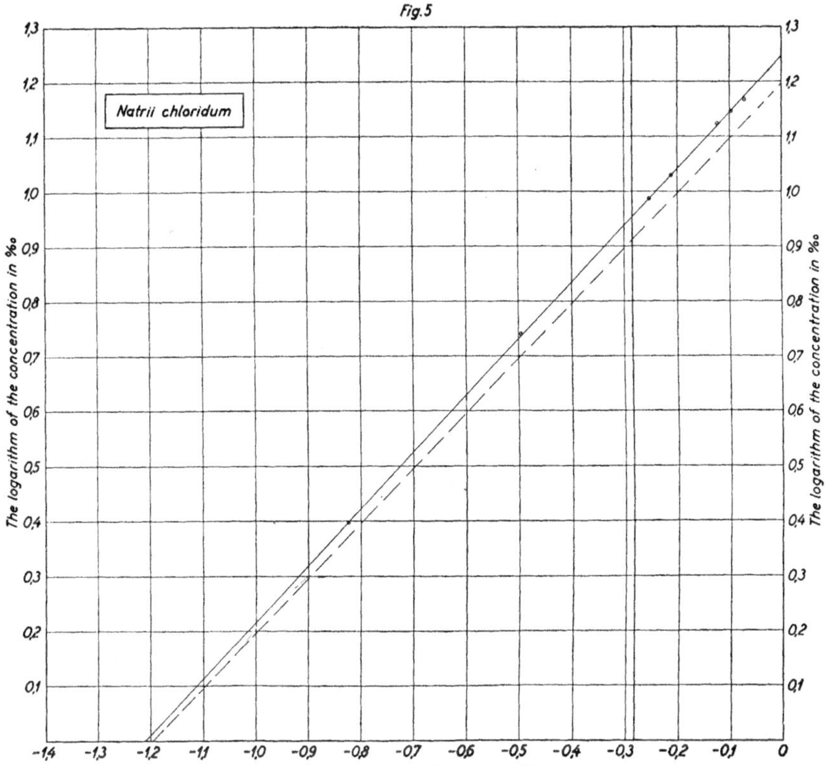

If, however, the system is to be used practically, it is much simpler to employ the arithmetical system, as the troublesome calculations then are avoided. The results obtained have, therefore,

Fig. 6

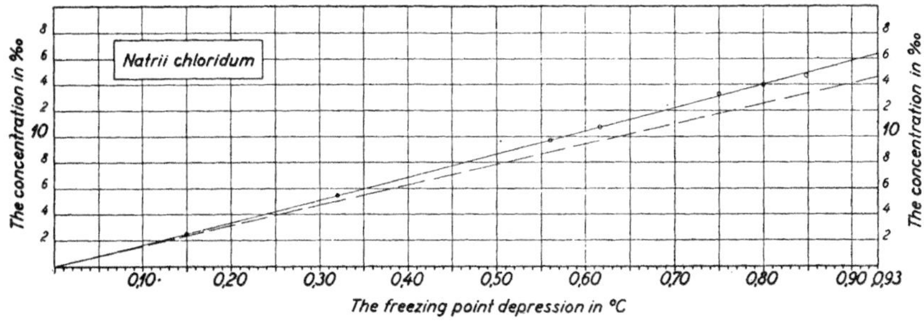

first been marked in the logarithmic system, the straight line has been drawn, and its equation calculated. Then this line has been transferred to the arithmetical system with so many points as are necessary to be able to draw the more or less arched curve, as will be seen in fig. 6.

In table 11 a comparison has been made between the sodium chloride values found by other authors, and our own values.

It will be seen that in table 11 there is a good agreement between *Böhme*'s values and our own. In the case of *Ph. Helvet.* the remarkable thing is that 2 of the values agree well with ours, whereas the first of the three values differs about 8 % from our value. As mentioned, the values in *Ph. Helvet.* have been taken from a work by *Lumiére & Chevrotier.* It is probable that these research

Table 11.

Author	The concentration expressed in ‰	The freezing point depression	The freezing point depression we find according to fig. 6
Brit. Pharm. Codex 1934	9.1	0.56	0.526
» » »	10.0	0.585	0.576
» » »	14.0	0.86	0.799
Böhme	3.4	0.200	0.202
»	6.8	0.400	0.396
»	13.8	0.800	0.788
Ph. Helvet.	9.0	0.560	0.520
»	10.0	0.585	0.576
»	14.0	0.800	0.799
Rosenthaler	9.0	0.560	0.520
»	14.0	0.800	0.799
Warburg	4.39	0.265	0.259
»	8.77	0.523	0.508
»	13.15	0.772	0.752

workers have found the values for 14 and 10 ‰ themselves, but as regards the values of a 9 ‰ sodium chloride solution it may be that they have not wanted to reject the prevailing statement that the latter solution should correspond to a freezing point depression of 0.56°.

No doubt this figure has become the result because no correction of the determinations has been made. If this correction is made, by weighing the amount of disengaged ice, it is found (as seen in fig. 4) that a sodium chloride solution of 9 ‰ has a freezing point depression not of 0.56°, but of 0.52°.

There is likewise a fair agreement between *Warburg*'s values and our own. *Warburg* also states to have corrected his result according to the amount of disengaged ice.

Furthermore we have compared our determinations with the values of 2 tables in *Landolt-Börnstein*. It proved that these values, too, represented a straight line in the logarithmic system, but with the inclination a = 1.0173, where we find a = 1.03. And F was 0.53°, if K was 9, where we find F = 0.52°, if K = 9.

5. *Results.*

In the following tables (12—48) the results determined have been stated, each substance in its own table. The substances have been given in the order in which they enter the accompanying figures. In most cases the results have been reached by determination of the vapour pressure of the solutions, which has then been changed into the corresponding freezing point depression. In a few cases, where this was not possible, the result has been obtained by means of *Beckmann*'s thermometer. In cases where there are results stated in literature a comparison has been made of the results others have found with those obtained by us. In the accompanying figures the calculated and the experimental curves have been marked in pairs, so that a true estimate of the difference can be formed.

Acidum boricum.

Vapour pressure determinations were made of the following solutions of boric acid. In table 13 the results are given in the corresponding freezing point depressions.

Table 13.

The concentration of boric acid in ‰	3.33	6.65	13.30	26.60	30.00
The corresponding freezing point depression in °C.	0.100	0.197	0.388	0.676	0.794

The equation of boric acid is: $K = 37.85 \cdot F^{1.0515}$.

The values stated in table 13 are the results of determinations of boric acid solutions, which have been sterilized under pressure. It is a strange fact that a newly prepared solution of boric acid that has been made without the application of heat gives a somewhat greater freezing point depression than after a heat treatment. For instance a newly prepared solution of 2.85 % and a 3.1 % solution which had been sterilized under pressure both showed a freezing point depression of 0.82°.

In table 14 a comparison has been made between the boric acid values of others and our own values.

As will be seen, the agreement is best with *Schou*'s value. There is also a good agreement with the freezing point depression of a 31 ‰ solution of boric acid in *Ph. Helvet.*, whereas the values for 10 and 22 ‰ solution of boric acid differ 12 % and 6 % respectively from our values. The values in *Ph. Helvet.* are all lower than ours, whereas *Henrioul*'s and *Rosenthaler*'s are higher, and they do not differ much from the theoretically calculated values. Possibly this may be due to the fact that the two latter authors have determined newly prepared solutions, and not solutions that have been sterilized under pressure.

Table 14.

Author	The concentration in ‰	The freezing point depression	The freezing point depression we find according to fig. 7
Henrioul	25.0	0.755	0.675
Ph. Helvet.	10.0	0.250	0.283
»	22.0	0.560	0.598
»	31.0	0.800	0.821
Rosenthaler	27.5	0.800	0.735
Schou	10.0	0.277	0.283
Own result	19.0		0.520

Atropini sulfas.

Vapour pressure determinations were made of the following solutions of atropine sulphate. In table 15 the results have been given in the corresponding freezing point depressions.

Table 15.

The concentration of atropine sulphate in ‰	5.00	10.00	20.00	100.0
The corresponding freezing point depression in °C.	0.041	0.073	0.123	0.581

The equation of the curve is: $K = 182.8 \cdot F^{1.11}$.

In table 16 a comparison is made between the atropine sulphate values of others, and our own values.

Table 16.

Author	The concentration in ‰	The freezing point depression	The freezing point depression we find according to fig. 7
Brit. Pharm. Codex 1934 and Ph. Helvet.	10.0	0.074	0.073
Rosenthaler	75.5	0.56	0.451
»	108.0	0.80	0.622
Schou	10.0	0.086	0.073
Own result	88.5		0.520

It will be seen from table 16, that while there is a good agreement between the *Ph. Helvet.* values and ours, there is a great divergency between *Rosenthaler*'s and *Schou*'s values on one hand and, on the other hand, our own values. *Schou* finds that an atropine sulphate solution of 1 % should correspond to a sodium chloride solution of 0.14 %, which gives a freezing point depression of 0.086°, where we find 0.073°. We find the isoosmotic concentration to be 88.5 ‰, whereas *Rosenthaler* states it is 75.5 ‰.

Cocaini hydrochloridum.

Vapour pressure determinations were made of the following solutions of cocaine hydrochloride. In table 17 the results have been given in the corresponding freezing point depressions.

Table 17.

The concentration of cocaine hydrochloride in ‰	18.26	36.52	50.60	73.04
The corresponding freezing point depression in °C.	0.160	0.314	0.436	0.596

The equation of the curve is: $K = 126.0 \cdot F^{1.054}$.

In table 18 a comparison is made between the values of cocaine hydrochloride of others, and our own values.

Table 18.

Author	The concentration in ‰	The freezing point depression	The freezing point depression we find according to fig. 7
Brit. Pharm. Codex 1934 ..	10.00	0.120	0.090
Ph. Helvet.	10.00	0.120	0.090
»	30.00	0.350	0.256
»	60.00	0.560	0.494
Rosenthaler	60.00	0.560	0.494
»	80.00	0.800	0.650
Schou	10.00	0.086	0.090
Own result	63.3		0.520

It is evident from table 18 that there is a very great difference between our values and those stated by *Brit. Pharm. Codex, Ph. Helvet.* and *Rosenthaler*. In the case of the concentration of 10 and 30 ‰ our freezing point depressions are about 25 % lower. On the other hand, our freezing point depression of 0.090° is somewhat higher than the value stated by *Schou:* 0.086°. We find the isosmotic concentration to be 63.3 ‰.

Cupri sulfas.

Vapour pressure determinations were made of the following solutions of copper sulphate. In table 19 the results are given in the corresponding freezing point depressions.

Table 19.

The concentration of copper sulphate in ‰	20.00	40.00	80.00	100.0
The corresponding freezing point depression in °C.	0.179	0.326	0.590	0.743

The equation of the curve is: $K = 145.9 \cdot F^{1.156}$.

In table 20 a comparison has been made between the values of others and our own values.

It is seen from table 20 that there is a fairly good agreement between *Landolt-Börnstein*'s values and ours, the latter being 2 to 5 % higher; our lowest value is, however, 8 % higher than *Landolt-Börnstein*'s. *Rosenthaler*'s value, on the other hand, is no less than 33 % higher than our value; no doubt it has been calculated on the

Table 20.

Author	The concentration in ‰	The freezing point depression	The freezing point depression we find according to fig. 7
Landolt-Börnstein 1923	3.655	0.03791	0.041
» »	10.31	0.096	0.101
» »	25.00	0.212	0.217
» »	60.19	0.446	0.464
Ph. Helvet. and Remington	1.0	0.01	0.012
»	5.0	0.05	0.054
Rosenthaler	80.0	0.80	0.594
Own result	68.5		0.520

basis of the two values stated by *Ph. Helvet.* and *Remington.* But these values agree well with ours, and here we have an evident instance of the dangers of calculating the freezing point depression of a stronger concentration on the basis of the freezing point determination of a weaker concentration, since the curve, as is seen in figure 7, is not straight, but rather arched. It is only when the curve is straight, i. e. when the concentration and the freezing point depression are in a direct ratio within the whole of the area which is of practical use, that it will be possible to calculate accurately the freezing point depression that any concentration will show, the calculation being based on the knowledge of the freezing point depression that a given concentration shows.

Pilocarpini hydrochloridum.

Vapour pressure determinations were made of the following solutions of pilocarpine hydrochloride. The results are given in the corresponding freezing point depressions in table 21.

Table 21.

The concentration of pilocarpine hydrochloride in ‰	12.50	25.00	50.00
The corresponding freezing point depression in °C.	0.160	0.320	0.634

The equation of the curve is: $K = 79.14 \cdot F^{1.007}$.

In table 22 a comparison is made between the pilocarpine hydrochloride values of others, and our own values.

Table 22.

Author	The concentration in ‰	The freezing point depression	The freezing point depression we find according to fig. 7
Ph. Helvet.	30.00	0.420	0.387
Rosenthaler	49.00	0.560	0.621
»	70.50	0.800	0.891
Schou	10.00	0.120	0.128
Own result	40.8		0.520

In table 22 a certain agreement is seen with the value stated by *Schou*. On the other hand our values are about 11 % higher than *Rosenthaler*'s while our value for a 30 ‰ solution of pilocarpine hydrochloride is about 9 % lower than stated in *Ph. Helvet.* We find the isoosmotic concentration to be 40.8 ‰, whereas Rosenthaler's value is 49 ‰.

Zinci sulfas.

In the case of zinc sulphate we made partly determinations of the freezing point depression, partly vapour pressure determinations. The results are seen in table 23.

Table 23.

The concentration of zinc sulphate in ‰	The concentration corrected at the freezing point determinations	The corresponding freezing point depression	The vapour pressure determination changed into freezing point depression
5.00	5.30	0.058	
7.73			0.070
10.00	11.10	0.097	
10.00	11.20	0.098	
15.46			0.127
15.00	15.50	0.130	
20.00	20.60	0.170	
25.00	27.10	0.200	
30.92			0.232
30.00	32.40	0.235	
35.00	37.80	0.269	
40.00	43.20	0.303	
50.00			0.349
50.00	53.20	0.368	
61.84			0.421
100.0			0.677
100.0	104.8	0.703	

The equation of the curve is: $K = 159.1 \cdot F^{1.1186}$.

Table 23 and fig. 7 show that there is a very good relationship between the values found directly by means of the determination of the freezing point depression, and the values found indirectly by determination of the vapour pressure. It must be emphasized that this agreement has been reached even if the freezing point determinations were made at a temperature of 0°, and the vapour pressure determinations at 20°.

Zinc sulphate and sodium citrate are the only two substances examined in this treatise on which we have made determinations by both the freezing point depression and relative vapour pressure methods. The results in each case, however, show the justification of the correction for the amount of disengaged ice in the former method, and confirm the reliability of the latter method.

There is a great difference between our values and those in *Ph. Helvet.*, stating freezing point depressions of 0.015° and 0.070° in zinc sulphate solutions of 1 and 5 ‰ respectively, whereas we find 0.010° and 0.045° respectively for the same concentrations. *Rosenthaler*'s freezing point depression, however, of 0.800° for a 113 ‰ solution of zinc sulphate, is more probable. We find the isoosmotic concentration to be 76.5 ‰.

Henrioul calls attention to the fact that zinc sulphate was one of the first drugs to be used in the treatment of eye diseases, because of its antiseptic qualities. The application of it will, however, often be rather painful because of the acid reaction of the solution. It is for this reason that the pharmaceutical literature has several prescriptions for zinc eye drops, in which not only isoosmosis, but a neutral reaction have been obtained by adding sodium chloride and sodium citrate. See for example *Henrioul (1936)* and *Bijleveld & Dekking (1941)*.

In fig. 7 the values from tables 13, 15, 17, 19, 21, and 23 have been marked in the same manner as the values in fig. 6.

Alypini hydrochloridum.

Vapour pressure determinations were made of the following solutions of alypine hydrochloride. In table 24 the results are given in the corresponding freezing point depressions.

Table 24.

The concentration of alypine hydrochloride in ‰	12.50	25.00	60.00	75.00	85.00	100.0
The corresponding freezing point depression in °C. ..	0.156	0.294	0.534	0.638	0.686	0.810

Fig.7

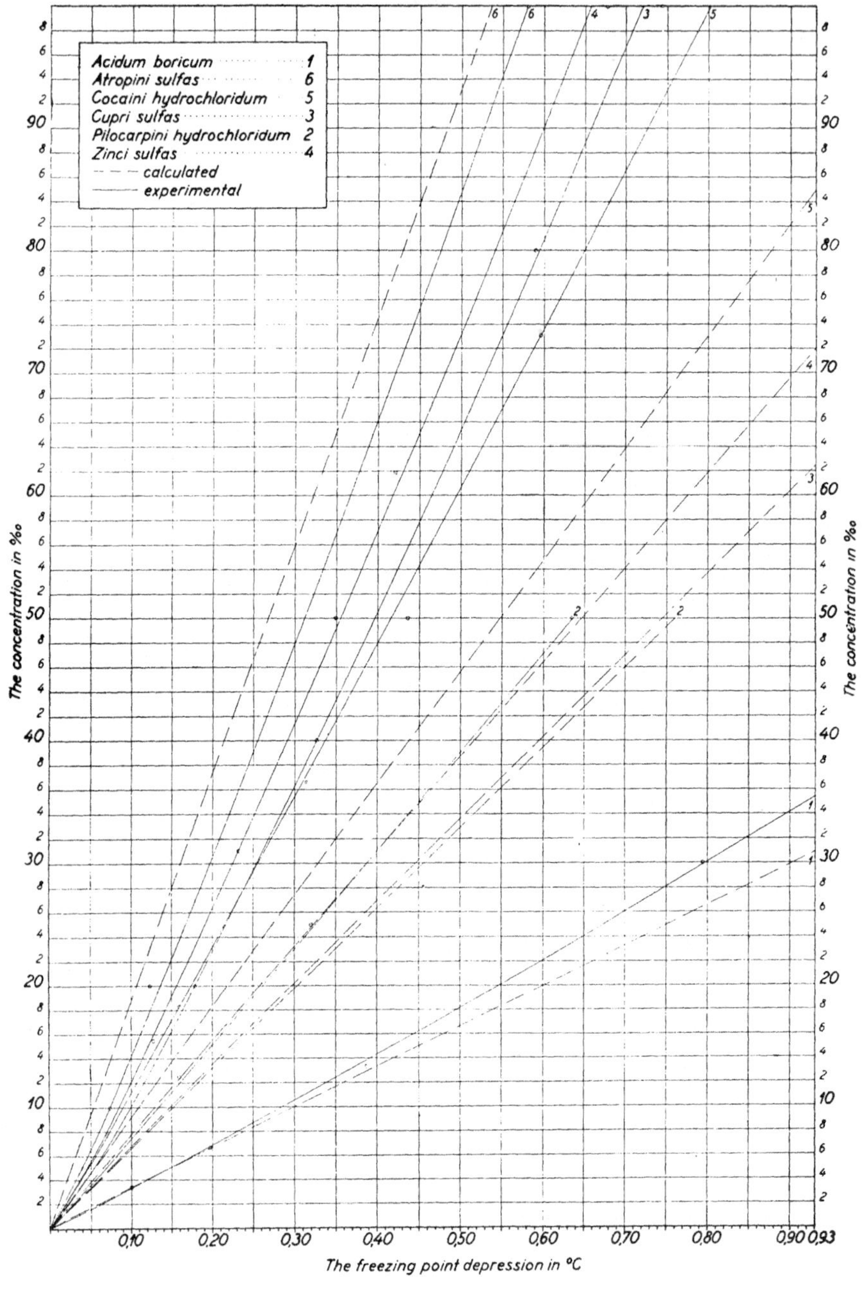
Acidum boricum 1
Atropini sulfas 6
Cocaini hydrochloridum 5
Cupri sulfas 3
Pilocarpini hydrochloridum 2
Zinci sulfas 4
calculated
experimental
The concentration in ‰
The freezing point depression in °C
0,10
0,20
0,30
0,40
0,50
0,60
0,70
0,80
0,90
0,93
10
20
30
40
50
60
70
80
90

The equation of the curve is: $K = 134.1 \cdot F^{1.301}$.

We have found no results in literature with which to compare our values.

Ephedrini hydrochloridum.

Vapour pressure determinations were made of the following solutions of ephedrine hydrochloride. In table 25 the results are given in the corresponding freezing point depressions.

Table 25.

The concentration of ephedrine hydrochloride in ‰	12.50	25.00	43.35	50.00
The corresponding freezing point depression in °C.	0.215	0.407	0.692	0.809

The equation of the curve is: $K = 62.55 \cdot F^{1.0186}$.

In table 26 a comparison is made between the ephedrine hydrochloride values of other authors, and our own values.

Table 26.

Author	The concentration in ‰	The freezing point depression	The freezing point depression we find according to fig. 8
Rosenthaler	40.50	0.56	0.656
»	58.00	0.80	0.933
Schou	10	0.162	0.169
Own result	32.0		0.520

It is evident from table 26 that there is a good agreement between *Schou*'s value and our own ones, but *Rosenthaler*'s freezing point depressions are about 13 or 14 % lower than our values. The isoosmotic concentration is stated by *Rosenthaler* to be 40.5 ‰, whereas we find it is 32.0 ‰.

Kalii chloras.

Vapour pressure determinations were made of the following solutions of potassium chlorate. In table 27 the results are given in the corresponding freezing point depressions.

Table 27.

The concentration of potassium chlorate in ⁰/₀₀	3.29	6.59	13.18	26.36	30.00
The corresponding freezing point depression in °C.	0.090	0.181	0.367	0.682	0.810

The equation of the curve is: $K = 36.67 \cdot F^{1.0053}$.

We have found no results in literature with which to compare our values.

Phenacainæ hydrochloridum.

Vapour pressure determinations were made of the following solutions of phenacaine hydrochloride (holocaine hydrochloride). In table 28 the results are given in the corresponding freezing point depressions.

Table 28.

The concentration of phenacaine hydrochloride in ⁰/₀₀	5.00	10.00	15.00
The corresponding freezing point depression in °C.	0.060	0.110	0.152

The equation of the curve is: $K = 148.0 \cdot F^{1.1211}$.

We have found no values in literature with which to compare our results.

Scopolamini hydrobromidum.

Vapour pressure determinations were made of the following solutions of scopolamine hydrobromide. In table 29 the results are given in the corresponding freezing point depressions.

Table 29.

The concentration of scopolamine hydrobromide in ⁰/₀₀	23.55	47.11	94.22	100.0
The corresponding freezing point depression in °C.	0.159	0.315	0.624	0.660

The equation of the curve is: $K = 152.1 \cdot F^{1.012}$.

There is a fine agreement with the value stated by *Schou,* that a 1 % solution of scopolamine hydrobromide should correspond to a 0.11 % solution of sodium chloride, which gives a freezing point depression of 0.068°. According to figure 8 we also get 0.068°.

In fig. 8 the values from tables 24, 25, 27, 28, and 29 have been marked in the same manner as the values in fig. 6.

Fig. 8

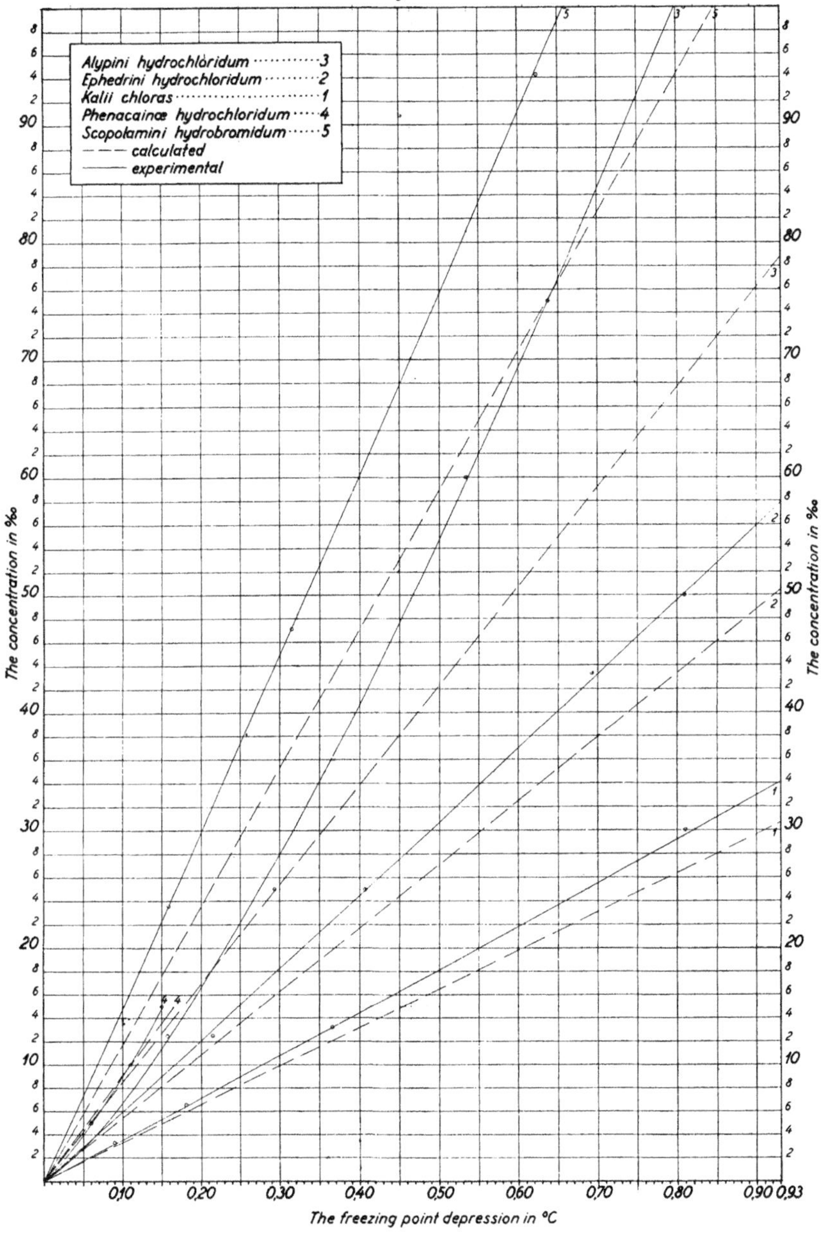
Alypini hydrochloridum 3
Ephedrini hydrochloridum 2
Kalii chloras 1
Phenacainæ hydrochloridum 4
Scopolamini hydrobromidum 5
calculated
experimental
The concentration in ‰
The freezing point depression in °C
0,10
0,20
0,30
0,40
0,50
0,60
0,70
0,80
0,90
0,93
10
20
30
40
50
60
70
80
90

Adrenalini bitartras.

Vapour pressure determinations were made of the following solutions of epinephrine bitartrate. In table 30 the results are given in the corresponding freezing point depressions.

Table 30.

The concentration of epinephrine bitartrate in ‰	6.25	12.50	25.00	50.00	75.00	100.0
The corresponding freezing point depression in °C.	0.062	0.121	0.226	0.475	0.674	0.900

The equation of the curve is: $K = 112.7 \cdot F^{1.040}$.

We have found no results in literature with which to compare our values.

Kalii nitras.

Vapour pressure determinations were made of the following solutions of potassium nitrate. In table 31 the results are given in the corresponding freezing point depressions.

Table 31.

The concentration of potassium nitrate in ‰	2.718	5.436	10.87	21.74	25.00
The corresponding freezing point depression in °C.	0.091	0.182	0.358	0.664	0.790

The equation of the potassium nitrate curve is: $K = 31.63 \cdot F^{1.02}$.

In table 32 a comparison is made between the values for potassium nitrate of others, and our own values.

Table 32.

Author	The concentration in ‰	The freezing point depression	The freezing point depression we find according to fig. 9
Brit. Pharm Codex 1934 ..	24.0	0.86	0.763
Böhme	5.9	0.200	0.202
»	12.4	0.400	0.400
»	19.0	0.600	0.635
»	26.0	0.800	0.864
Rosenthaler	26.0	0.800	0.864
Own result	16.2		0.520

It will be seen that while there is a good agreement between our values and those stated by *Böhme* and *Rosenthaler,* there is a great divergency between our value and the statement of *Brit. Pharm. Codex* for a 24.0 ‰ solution of potassium nitrate.

Methylatropini nitras.

Vapour pressure determinations were made of the following solutions of methylatropine nitrate. In table 33 the results are given in the corresponding freezing point depressions.

Table 33.

The concentration of methylatropine nitrate in ‰	12.50	25.00	50.00	100.0
The corresponding freezing point depression in °C.	0.119	0.225	0.412	0.743

The equation of the curve is: $K = 138.3 \cdot F^{1.147}$.

There is a great deviation from the value stated by *Schou* that a 1 % solution of methylatropine nitrate should correspond to a 0.14 % solution of sodium chloride, which gives a freezing point depression of 0.086°. According to fig. 9 we find 0.100°.

Natrii boras.

Vapour pressure determinations were made of the following solutions of sodium borate. In table 34 the results are given in the corresponding freezing point depressions.

Table 34.

The concentration of sodium borate in ‰	6.84	13.67	27.34	40.00	54.69
The corresponding freezing point depression in °C.	0.177	0.330	0.555	0.738	0.930

The equation of the curve is: $K = 58.25 \cdot F^{1.237}$.

There is a fairly good agreement between on one side our values and on the other side the freezing point depression of 0.220° for a 10 ‰ solution of sodium borate, as stated in *Ph. Helvet.* (where we find 0.24°). *Brit. Pharm. Codex* and *Rosenthaler,* stating freezing point depressions of 0.56° and 0.80° for solutions of sodium borate of 29.0 ‰ and 41.0 ‰ respectively. We find 0.57° and 0.75° respectively. According to fig. 9 the isoosmotic concentration is 26 ‰.

Physostigmini salicylas.

Vapour pressure determinations were made of the following solutions of physostigmine salicylate. In table 35 the results are given in the corresponding freezing point depressions.

Table 35.

The concentration of physostigmine salicylate in ‰	5.00	10.00
The corresponding freezing point depression in °C.	0.045	0.090

The equation of the curve is: $K = 11.9 \cdot F$.

Here the experimental and the theoretical values coincide. There is a great difference between our values and the value stated by *Schou*, saying that a 1 % solution of physostigmine salicylate should correspond to a 0.12 % solution of sodium chloride, which gives a freezing point depression of 0.073°. According to fig. 9 we find 0.090°. *Rosenthaler*'s value of 0.80° for a 17.8 % solution shows a great deviation from the curve resulting from the above equation. *Rosenthaler*'s value seems to be calculated from a determination of a much weaker solution, as the greatest concentration which it is possible to obtain in an aqueous solution of physostigmine salicylate is 10 ‰.

In fig. 9 the values from tables 30, 31, 33, 34, and 35 have been marked in the same manner as the values in fig. 6.

Aethylmorphini hydrochloridum.

Vapour pressure determinations were made of the following solutions of ethylmorphine hydrochloride. In table 36 the results are shown in the corresponding freezing point depressions.

Table 36.

The concentration of ethylmorphine hydrochloride in ‰	15.00	30.00	50.00	60.00
The corresponding freezing point depression in °C.	0.131	0.257	0.433	0.490

The equation of the curve is: $K = 120.9 \cdot F^{1.026}$.

There is a great difference between our values and *Schou*'s statement that a 1 % solution of ethylmorphine hydrochloride should correspond to an 0.12 % solution of sodium chloride, which gives a freezing point depression of 0.073°. According to fig. 10 we find 0.088°.

Fig. 9

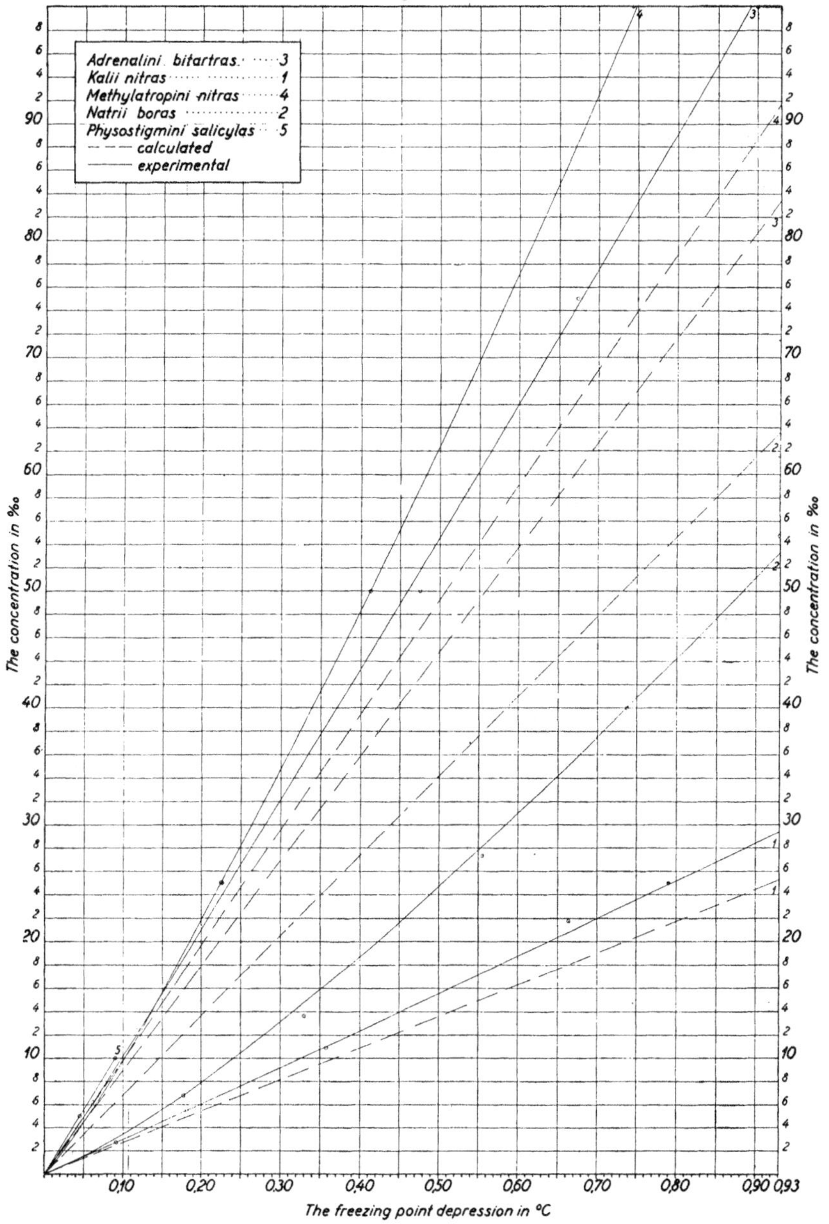
Adrenalini bitartras 3
Kalii nitras 1
Methylatropini nitras 4
Natrii boras 2
Physostigmini salicylas 5
calculated
experimental
The concentration in ‰
The freezing point depression in °C

Argenti nitras.

As mentioned before, the thermo-element in *Hill*'s apparatus is covered by an insulating coating of a special kind of varnish. Unfortunately it proved that this coating was not resistant to silver nitrate, which quickly penetrated it, and of course spoiled the thermo-element. So in the case of silver nitrate we had to make the test by a direct determination of the freezing point depression. The results, which have been corrected as to the amount of disengaged ice, are seen in table 37.

Table 37.

The concentration of silver nitrate in ⁰/₀₀	9.13	12.27	36.54
The corrected concentration	9.78	19.55	39.10
The corresponding freezing point depression in °C.	0.185	0.370	0.741

The equation of the silver nitrate curve is: $K = 52.70 \cdot F$.

In table 38 a comparison is made between the values for silver nitrate of other authors, and our own values.

Table 38.

Author	The concentration in ⁰/₀₀	The freezing point depression	The freezing point depression according to fig. 10
Brit. Pharm. Codex 1934 ..	10.0	0.20	0.190
Böhme	9.80	0.200	0.186
»	20.5	0.400	0.389
»	31.7	0.600	0.600
»	43.1	0.800	0.818
Landolt-Börnstein 1931	3.982	0.0810	0.076
»	6.378	0.1310	0.121
»	12.037	0.2402	0.229
»	23.925	0.4615	0.453
»	32.771	0.6163	0.618
Rosenthaler	43.0	0.800	0.815
Own result	27.4		0.520

It will be seen from Table 38 that there is a good agreement between *Brit. Pharm. Codex, Böhme's, Landolt-Börnstein*'s and our values in the cases of higher concentrations, whereas our freezing point depressions are somewhat lower for the lower concentrations.

Argyrol and Targesin.

Direct determinations of the freezing point were made of the following solutions of argyrol and targesin. The results are seen in table 39 and table 40 respectively.

Table 39.

The concentration of argyrol in ‰	25.00	25.00	50.00	50.00	100.0	100.0
The corrected concentration..	26.2	26.5	52.5	53.5	105.0	107.0
The corresponding freezing point depression in °C. ..	0.240	0.250	0.490	0.510	0.975	1.025

Table 40.

The concentration of targesin in ‰	25.00	25.00	50.00	50.00	100.0	100.0
The corrected concentration	26.3	26.5	53.0	53.5	105.0	105.5
The corresponding freezing point depression in °C. ..	0.240	0.250	0.510	0.510	0.988	1.020

It will be seen from tables 39 and 40 that argyrol and targesin show the same conditions, and therefore only one curve has been composed, which is representative of either substance, based on the following average values (Table 41).

Table 41.

The concentration of argyrol and targesin in ‰	26.38	53.40	105.9
The corresponding freezing point depression in °C.	0.245	0.504	1.002

The equation of the curve is: $K = 105.9 \cdot F$.

We have found no statements in literature, concerning the osmotic pressure of argyrol or targesin in aqueous solutions. It will be seen that a solution of 5 % will be nearly isoosmotic with lachrymal fluid. So weaker solutions ought to be adjusted by means of sodium nitrate in the same way as solutions of silver nitrate. Repeated determinations proved that such adjusted solutions preserved their osmotic qualities unchanged for three months.

Resorcinum.

Vapour pressure determinations were made of the following solutions of resorcinol. In table 42 the results are given in the corresponding freezing point depressions.

Table 42.

The concentration of resorcinol in ‰	8.70	12.50	17.50	25.00	35.00	47.33	50.0
The corresponding freezing point depression in °C.	0,141	0.202	0.281	0.402	0.546	0.724	0.770

The equation of the curve is: $K = 64.45 \cdot F^{1.023}$.

There is a good agreement between our values and those given by *Landolt-Börnstein,* who gives freezing point depressions of 0.229°, 0.446°, and 0.861° for resorcinol solutions of 13.9 ‰, 28.12 ‰, and 57.55 ‰ respectively. According to fig. 10 the isoosmotic concentration is 33 ‰.

Tropacocaini hydrochloridum.

Vapour pressure determinations were made of the following solutions of tropacocaine hydrochloride. In table 43 the results are given in the corresponding freezing point depressions.

Table 43.

The concentration of tropacocaine hydrochloride in ‰	12.50	25.00	50.00	75.00	100.0
The corresponding freezing point depression in °C.	0.162	0.302	0.531	0.726	0.882

The equation of the curve is: $K = 110.8 \cdot F^{1.238}$.

We have found no statements in literature, with which to compare our results.

In fig. 10 the values from tables 35, 37, 41, 42, and 43 have been marked in the same manner as the values in fig. 6.

Adrenoni hydrochloridum.

Vapour pressure determinations were made of the following solutions of adrenone hydrochloride. In table 44 the results are given in the corresponding freezing point depressions.

Table 44.

The concentration of adrenone hydrochloride in °C.	6.25	12.50	25.00	50.00	75.00
The corresponding freezing point depression in °C.	0.091	0.190	0.333	0.576	0.843

Fig. 10

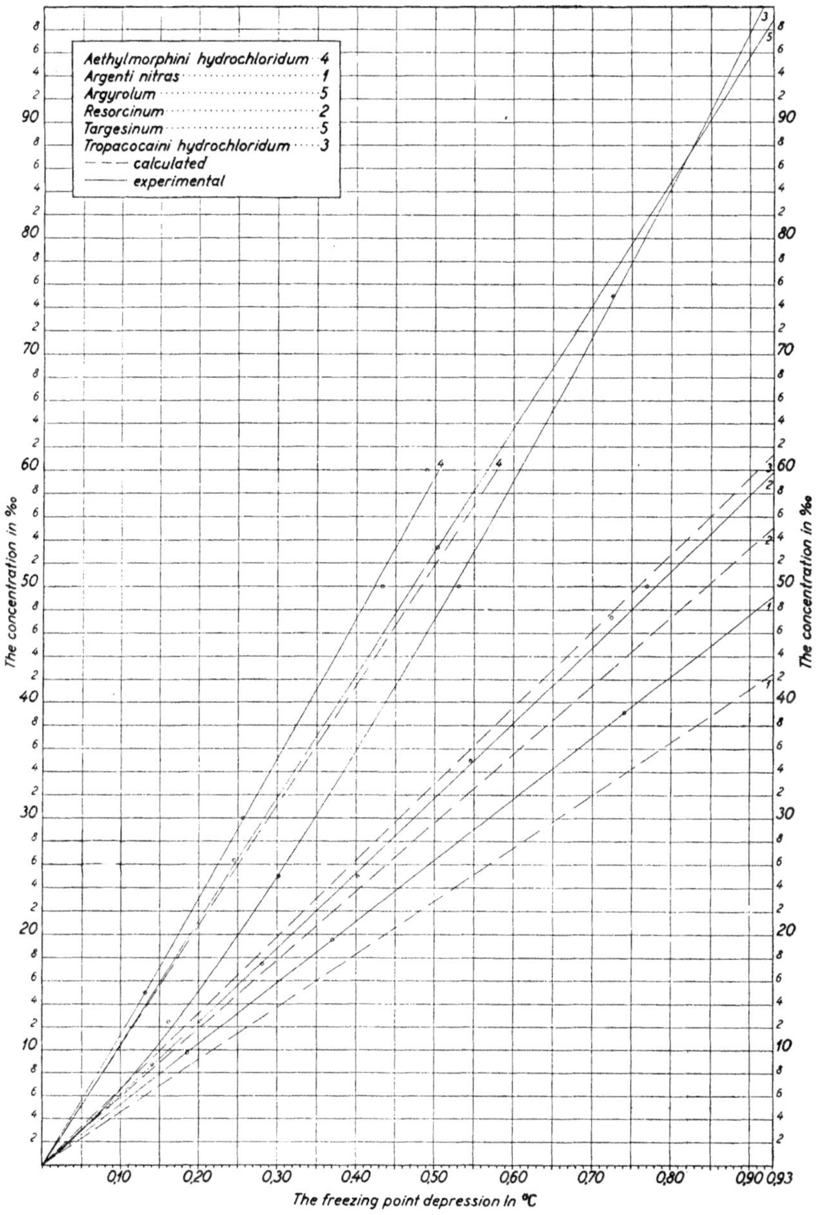

Aethylmorphini hydrochloridum 4
Argenti nitras 1
Argyrolum 5
Resorcinum 2
Targesinum 5
Tropacocaini hydrochloridum 3
calculated
experimental
The concentration in ‰
The freezing point depression In °C
0,10
0,20
0,30
0,40
0,50
0,60
0,70
0,80
0,90
0,93
10
20
30
40
50
60
70
80
90

The equation of the curve is: $K = 91.79 \cdot F^{1.184}$.

We have found no results in literature, with which to compare our results.

Aluminii kalii sulfas.

Vapour pressure determinations were made of the following solutions of potash alum. In table 45 the results are given in the corresponding freezing point depressions.

Table 45.

The concentration of potash alum in ‰	8.50	17.00	34.00	68.09	85.00
The corresponding freezing point depression in °C.	0.080	0.161	0.294	0.550	0.668

The equation of the curve is: $K = 133.6 \cdot F^{1.126}$.

We are in complete agreement with the freezing point depression of 0.100° for a 10 ‰ solution of potash alum, as stated in *Brit. Pharm. Codex* and *Ph. Helvet.*, as we find exactly the same value. But *Rosenthaler*'s value of 0.80° in the case of a 86.5 ‰ solution of potash alum differs much from our value: 0.678°. According to fig. 11 the isoosmotic concentration is 63.5 ‰.

Fluoresceinnatrium.

Vapour pressure determinations were made of the following solutions of soluble fluorescein. In table 46 the results are given in the corresponding freezing point depressions.

Table 46.

The concentration of soluble flourescein in ‰	6.25	12.50	25.00	50.00
The corresponding freezing point depression in °C.	0.121	0.220	0.407	0.732

The equation of the curve is: $K = 71.35 \cdot F^{1.152}$.

We have found no values in literature, with which to compare our results.

Homatropini hydrobromidum.

Vapour pressure determinations were made of the following solutions of homatropine hydrobromide. In table 47 the results are given in the corresponding freezing point depressions.

Table 47.

The concentration of homatropine hydrobromide in ‰	19.15	38.29	50.00	76.58	100.0
The corresponding freezing point depression in °C.	0.180	0.355	0.460	0.685	0.892

The equation of the curve is: $K = 110.6 \cdot F^{1.026}$.

There is a very great difference between *Schou*'s statement, saying that a 1% solution of homatropine hydrobromide should correspond to a 0.13 % solution of sodium chloride, which gives a freezing point depression of 0.079°, and our value according to fig. 11: 0.096°. The same is the case with *Rosenthaler*'s value of 0.800° for a 10.25 % solution of homatropine hydrobromide, where we find 0.929°.

Optochini hydrochloridum.

Vapour pressure determinations were made of the following solutions of ethylhydrocupreine hydrochloride. In table 48 the results are given in the corresponding freezing point depressions.

Table 48.

The concentration af ethylhydrocupreine hydrochloride in ‰	6.25	12.50	25.00	50.00	60.00	75.00	85.00	100.0
The corresponding freezing point depression in °C.	0.073	0.112	0.180	0.270	0.302	0.316	0.339	0.353

The equation of the curve for solutions up to 60 ‰ is:
$K = 403.6 \cdot F^{1.592}$.

We have found no statements in literature, with which to compare our results.

Some peculiar facts about the values for ethylhydrocupreine hydrochloride are worth mentioning. In the *logarithmic* system the values amounting to concentrations up to 60 ‰ lie on a straight line, which cuts the ordinate at an angle of a little less than 45°. For concentrations stronger than 60 ‰ the determined values lie on a straight line, too, but the latter line has a still steeper course, and forms a still smaller angle with the ordinate. In the *arithmetical* system in fig. 11 there is no great difference between the freezing point depressions caused by ethylhydrocupreine hydrochloride solutions of 60 ‰ and 100 ‰ (see table 48).

In fig. 11 the values from tables 44, 45, 46, 47, and 48 have been marked in the same manner as the values in fig. 6.

Fig.11

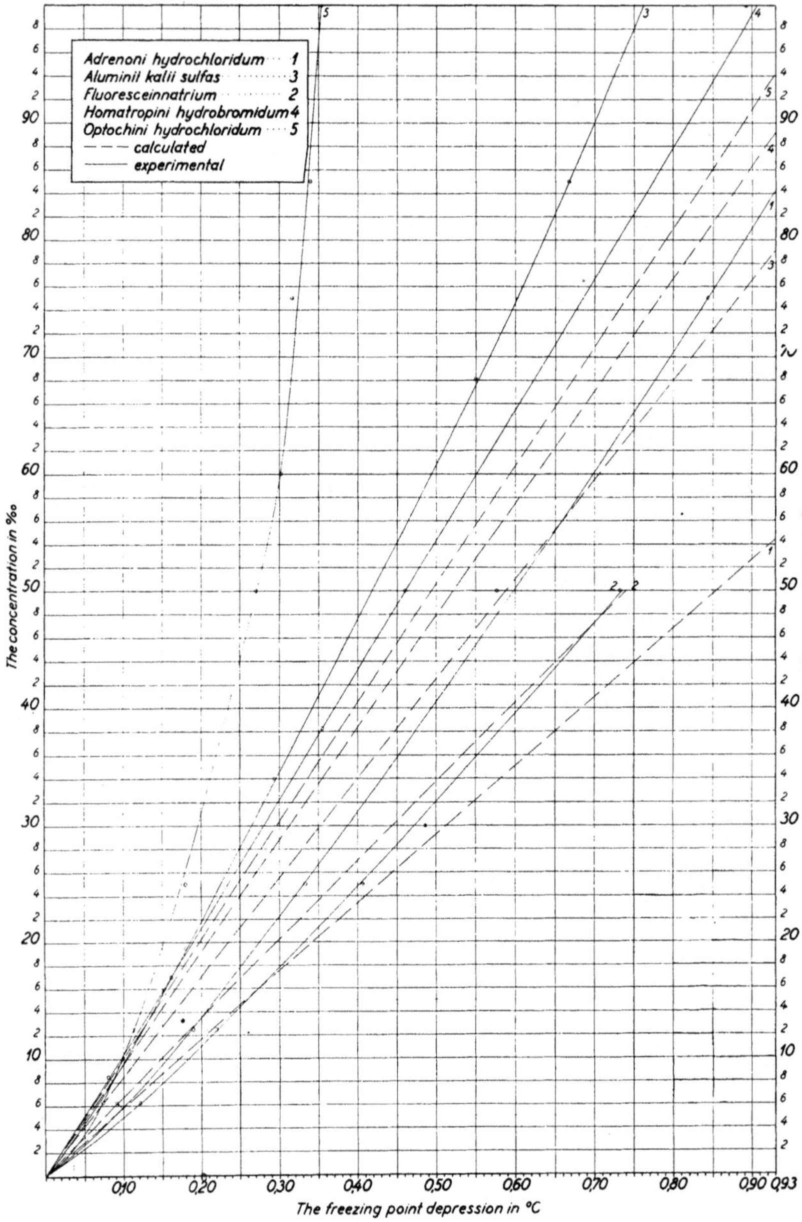

Adrenoni hydrochloridum 1
Aluminii kalii sulfas 3
Fluoresceinnatrium 2
Homatropini hydrobromidum 4
Optochini hydrochloridum 5
calculated
experimental
The concentration in ‰
The freezing point depression in °C
0,10
0,20
0,30
0,40
0,50
0,60
0,70
0,80
0,90
0,93
10
20
30
40
50
60
70
80
90

6. Activity relations.

It will be seen from figures 7—11 that generally there is never agreement between the calculated and the experimentally found values. As mentioned before, this is due to the activity relations of the solutions. It is of interest to look more closely into the activities that have been stated in our material. It must be noted that the activity coefficients stated in this section result from a comparison of the freezing point depressions calculated in the customary manner (where the concentration has been expressed in w/v), and the experimentally found freezing point depressions, (where, in view of the practical work involved in the preparation of eye drops, w/w concentrations have been used).

As mentioned before, an ideal 1-molar solution of a substance which has not been dissociated gives a freezing point depression of 1.86° (1.858°). If the substance is dissociated in 2 ions the results is 3.72°, and for a substance which is dissociated in 3 ions the result is 5.580°.

In case	I	a	1-molar	solution	will	be	1-osmolar
» »	II	»	½-molar	»	»	»	1-osmolar
	and	»	1-molar	»	»	»	2-osmolar
» »	III	»	⅓-molar	»	»	»	1-osmolar
	and	»	1-molar	»	»	»	3-osmolar

If the values for the freezing point depression of 1.86° had been included on the abscissa of the figures, the 1-molar concentrations for all the substances might have been read directly at the same time. We have, however, drawn a thick line, representing a freezing point depression of 0.93°, so that the semiosmolar concentrations can be read directly from our figures.

Looking at the curves for sodium chloride it is found that a 1.48 % solution, calculated by equation II, is to bring about a freezing point depression of 0.93°, whereas, according to the curve of the experimental determinations, a 1.48 % solution only gives a freezing point depression of 0.83°. The activity coefficient (f) in this case is 0.83/0.93 = 0.892.

By means of the calculated and experimental curves shown in figures 7—11 we have in table 49 made some calculations of activity coefficients for solutions of the substances in question, which give freezing point depressions of 0.186°, 0.52°, and 0.93°, in so far as it has been possible to prepare solutions of the necessary concentrations.

Table 49.

The name of the substance	Freezing point depression		
	0.186	0.52	0.93
	The activity coefficient f		
Acidum boricum	0.953	0.911	0.873
Adrenalini bitartras	0.846	0.817	
Adrenoni hydrochloridum	0.871	0.715	0.648
Aethylmorphini hydrochloridum	0.897	0.872	
Aluminii kalii sulfas	0.790	0.663	
Alypini hydrochloridum	1.033	0.765	
Argenti nitras	0.866	0.866	0.866
Atropini sulfas	1.238	1.095	
Cocaini hydrochloridum	0.785	0.748	
Cupri sulfas	0.590	0.510	
Ephedrini hydrochloridum	0.893	0.881	0.872
Fluoresceinnatrium	1.225	1.045	
Homatropini hydrochloridum	0.904	0.880	0.869
Kalii chloras	0.910	0.900	0.900
Kalii nitras	0.893	0.870	0.861
Metylatropini nitras	0.901	0.784	
Natrii boras (n = 3)	1.750	1.365	1.193
Natrii boras (n = 4)	1.306	1.025	0.895
Natrii chloridum	0.935	0.906	0.892
Optochini hydrochloridum	0.680		
Pilocarpini hydrochloridum	0.864	0.840	
Resorcinum	0.957	0.930	0.921
Scopolamini hydrobromidum	0.794	0.786	
Tropacocaini hydrochloridum	0.884	0.693	0.603
Zinci sulfas	0.588	0.520	

It will be seen that two activity coefficients have been calculated for natrii boras. The results we have found indicate that we were wrong when we took it for granted that sodium borate was ionized in three ions. So it is possible that the borate is dissociated in aqueous solution in a manner different from the one generally used for calculation.

7. Control of the eye drops in Dispensatorium Danicum.

Based on the present material we have made a review of the eye drops embodied in D. D. 1938, and rendered an account of this review in table 50 (see below).

The proposals in the last column have all been prepared and thoroughly tested and found isoosmotic.

In Pharmaconomia Svecica II, 1943 there are a great number of

Table 50.

Oculoguttae	Adjusted by addition of:	The composition which would have correspon- ded to 1.4 % of NaCl	The compo- sition which corresponds to 0.9 % of NaCl
aethylmorphini	1.15 % of NaCl	as in D. D. 1938	0.65 % of NaCl
argenti nitratis	2.02 % » KNO_3	» » » »	1.20 % » KNO_3
atropini	1.35 % » NaCl	» » » »	0.85 % » NaCl
cocaini	1.10 % » NaCl	» » » »	0.60 % » NaCl
homatropini	1.35 % » NaCl	» » » »	0.85 % » NaCl
physostigmini	1.30 % » NaCl	1.25 % of NaCl	0.75 % » NaCl
pilocarpini	1.00 % » NaCl	0.95 % of NaCl	0.50 % » NaCl
scopolamini	1.40 % » NaCl	as in D. D. 1938	0.90 % » NaCl
zinci sulfatis	1.35 % » NaCl	» » » »	0.85 % » NaCl
zinci sulfatis boricae	2.00 % » H_3BO_3	2.65 % of H_3BO_3	1.70 % » H_3BO_3

prescriptions for eye drops. They are fixed at such a concentration as to be isoosmotic with a 1.4 % solution of sodium chloride. Those of the eye drops that have the same names as the corresponding solutions in D. D. nearly all of them contain larger amounts of the active substance than the Danish ones, so we have not seen occasion to discuss them here.

8. *Eye lotions.*

In D. D. 1938 there are two prescriptions for eye lotions: Aqua ophthalmica boraxata and Solutio hydrargyri oxycyanidi.

As it must be supposed that the correct osmotic concentration is of at least as great an importance to eye lotions as to eye drops we have examined the two eye lotions mentioned above.

Aqua ophthalmica boraxata:

According to the curve in fig. 9, a 1 % solution of sodium borate indicates a freezing point depression of 0.24°. So it is very hypoosmotic. An isoosmotic solution must contain 2.6 % of sodium borate. By analogy to the pH for eye drops, (which we have already mentioned in this treatise) an eye lotion, in the application of which it is intended to change the pH of the mucous membranes towards alkalinity, ought not (according to *Hosforth & Hicks* (1935)) to be more alkaline than pH 7.35, but should contain a buffer-mixture which can fix this natural acidity in the diseased eye. A solution, sterilized under pressure, and containing 0.25 % of sodium borate and 1.75 % of boric acid will have a pH about 7.35 and be isoosmotic with a 9 ‰ sodium chloride solution. If the freezing point depression of this solution is to be calculated by adding together the values for boric acid and sodium borate on the basis of figures 7 and 9 the result will be 0.56°, and not 0.52°. This disagreement is possibly due to the fact that boric acid and sodium borate in an aqueous solution affect each other as to the total activity.

In *Pharmaconomia Svecica II (1943)* we find Aqua ophthalmica borata containing 1.33 % of sodium borate and 2.00 % of boric acid in distilled water.

Solutio hydrargyri oxycyanidi is very hypotonic. It has been attempted to make the solution isoosmotic by adding sodium cloride, but this makes the solution very alkaline. *Henrioul* finds the pH to be 10.73. So, in addition to sodium chloride, *Henrioul* proposes to add so much boric acid as to obtain an almost neutral reaction. This is basically unsound, as a solution of mercuric chloride-sodium chloride might then have been used instead. Here we propose either to dissolve the mercuric oxycyanide in an Aqua ophthalmica boraxata of the composition proposed above (0.25 % of sodium borate and 1.75 % of boric acid), or to make the adjustment by means of potassium nitrate; 1.62 % of this substance is then to be added.

9. Summary.

Freezing point determinations and determinations of the relative vapour pressure have been made of aqueous solutions of substances that are used in the preparation of eye drops. The results have been entered into a system of coordinates in figures 12, 13, 14, 15, and 16. It is proposed to employ this system of coordinates in a future Danish pharmacopoeia for use at the preparation of extemporaneously prescribed eye drops, so that these can be isoosmotic with lachrymal fluid. It is also proposed to prepare eye lotions according to the same rules.

Fig.12

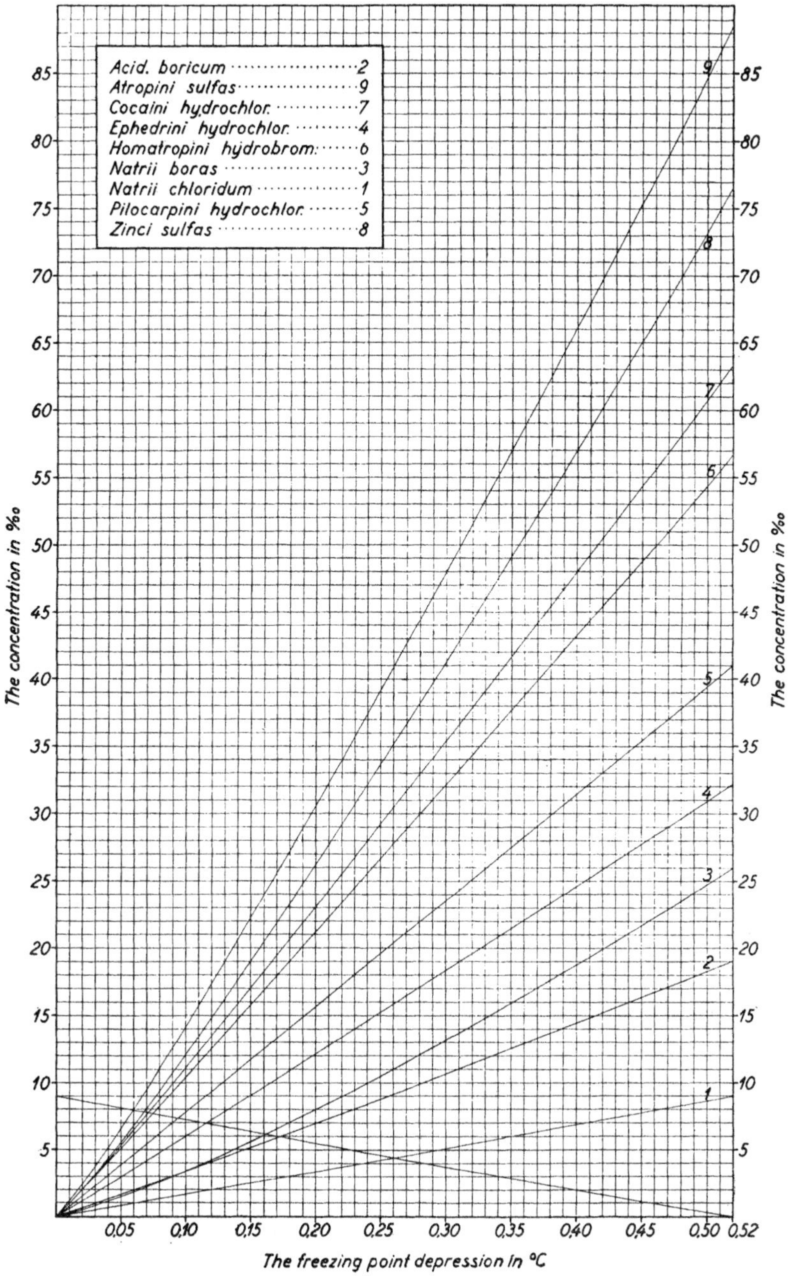

Acid. boricum 2
Atropini sulfas 9
Cocaini hydrochlor. 7
Ephedrini hydrochlor. 4
Homatropini hydrobrom. 6
Natrii boras 3
Natrii chloridum 1
Pilocarpini hydrochlor. 5
Zinci sulfas 8
The concentration in ‰
The freezing point depression in °C
0,05 0,10 0,15 0,20 0,25 0,30 0,35 0,40 0,45 0,50 0,52
5 10 15 20 25 30 35 40 45 50 55 60 65 70 75 80 85

Fig.13

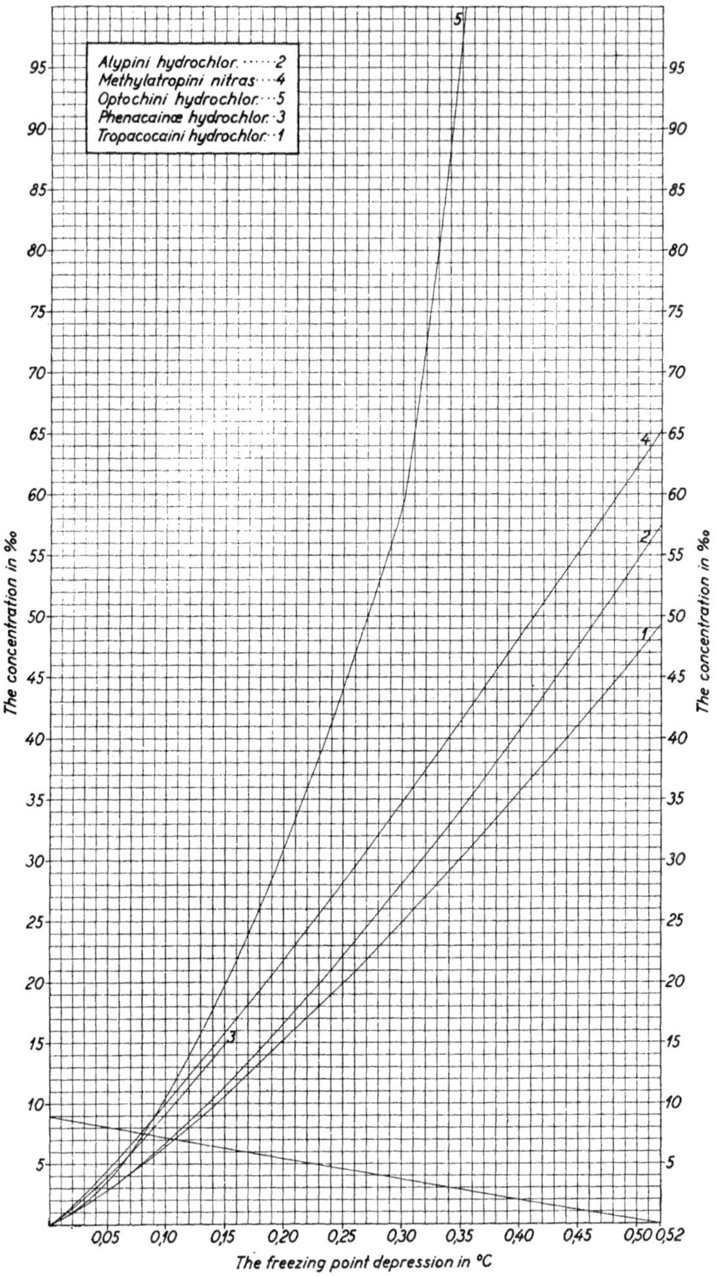
Alypini hydrochlor. ······2
Methylatropini nitras ···4
Optochini hydrochlor. ···5
Phenacainæ hydrochlor. ·3
Tropacocaini hydrochlor. ·1
The concentration in ‰
The freezing point depression in °C
0,05 0,10 0,15 0,20 0,25 0,30 0,35 0,40 0,45 0,50 0,52
5 10 15 20 25 30 35 40 45 50 55 60 65 70 75 80 85 90 95

Fig. 14

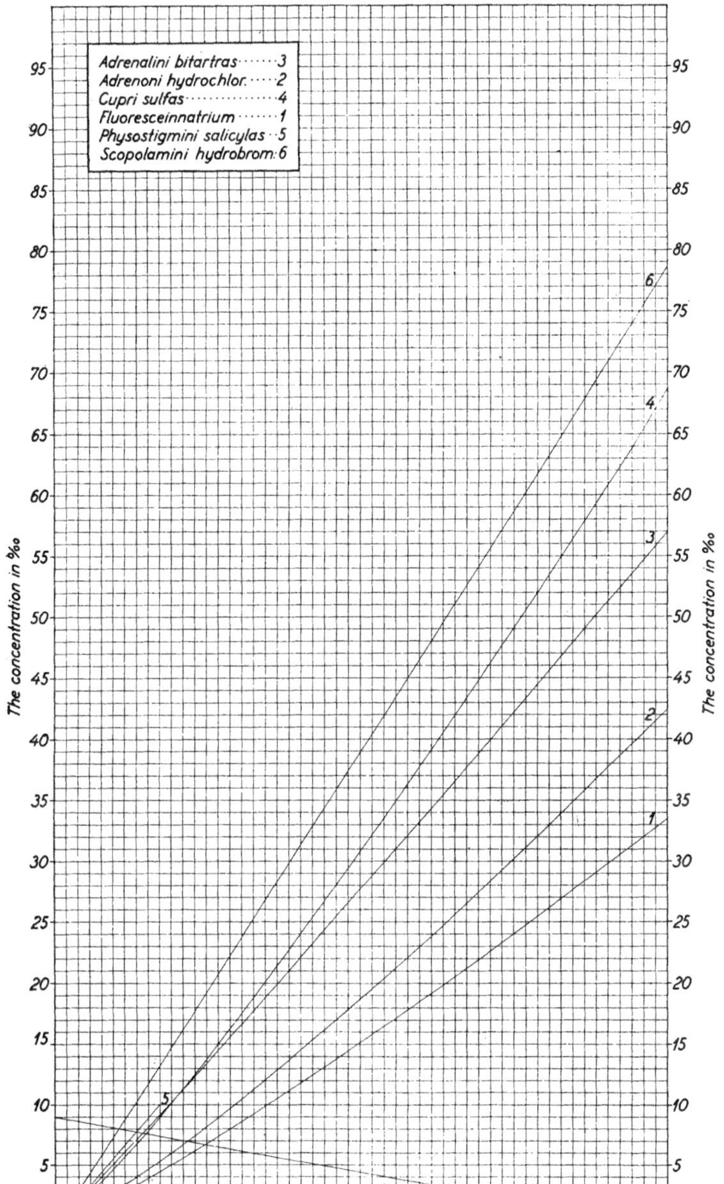
Adrenalini bitartras 3
Adrenoni hydrochlor. 2
Cupri sulfas 4
Fluoresceinnatrium 1
Physostigmini salicylas .. 5
Scopolamini hydrobrom. 6
The concentration in ‰
The freezing point depression in °C
95
90
85
80
75
70
65
60
55
50
45
40
35
30
25
20
15
10
5
0,05 0,10 0,15 0,20 0,25 0,30 0,35 0,40 0,45 0,50 0,52
6
4
3
2
1
5

Fig. 15

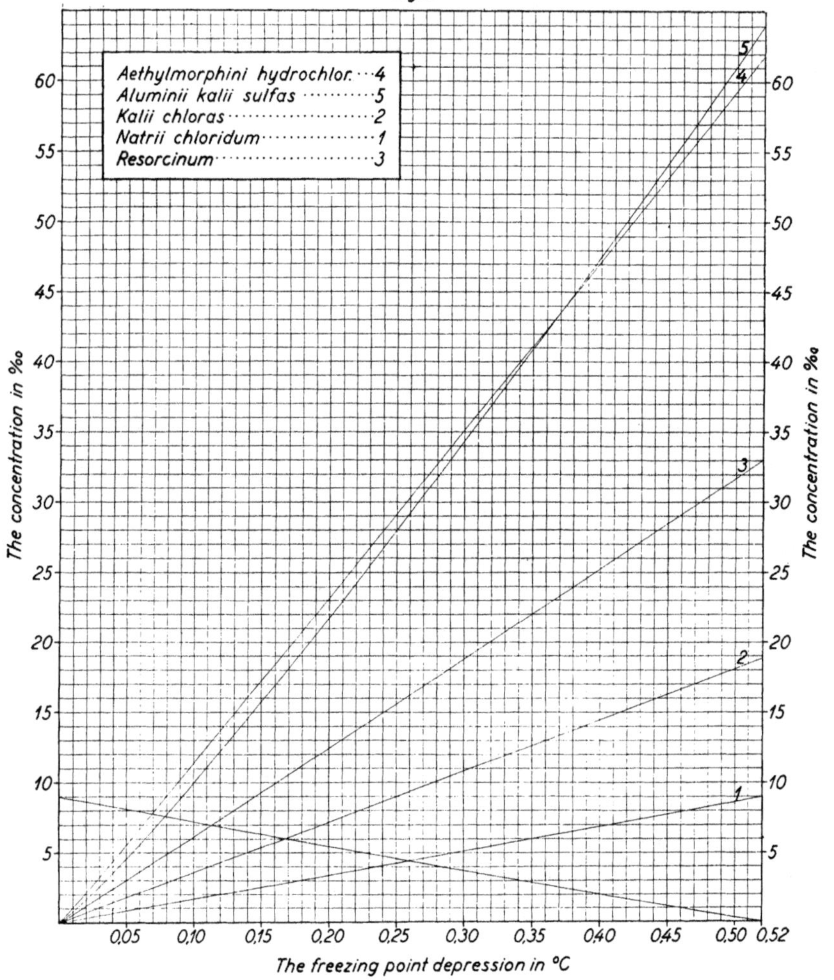

Aethylmorphini hydrochlor. ··· 4
Aluminii kalii sulfas ········· 5
Kalii chloras ················· 2
Natrii chloridum ·············· 1
Resorcinum ···················· 3
The concentration in ‰
The freezing point depression in °C
60
55
50
45
40
35
30
25
20
15
10
5
0,05 0,10 0,15 0,20 0,25 0,30 0,35 0,40 0,45 0,50 0,52

Fig. 16

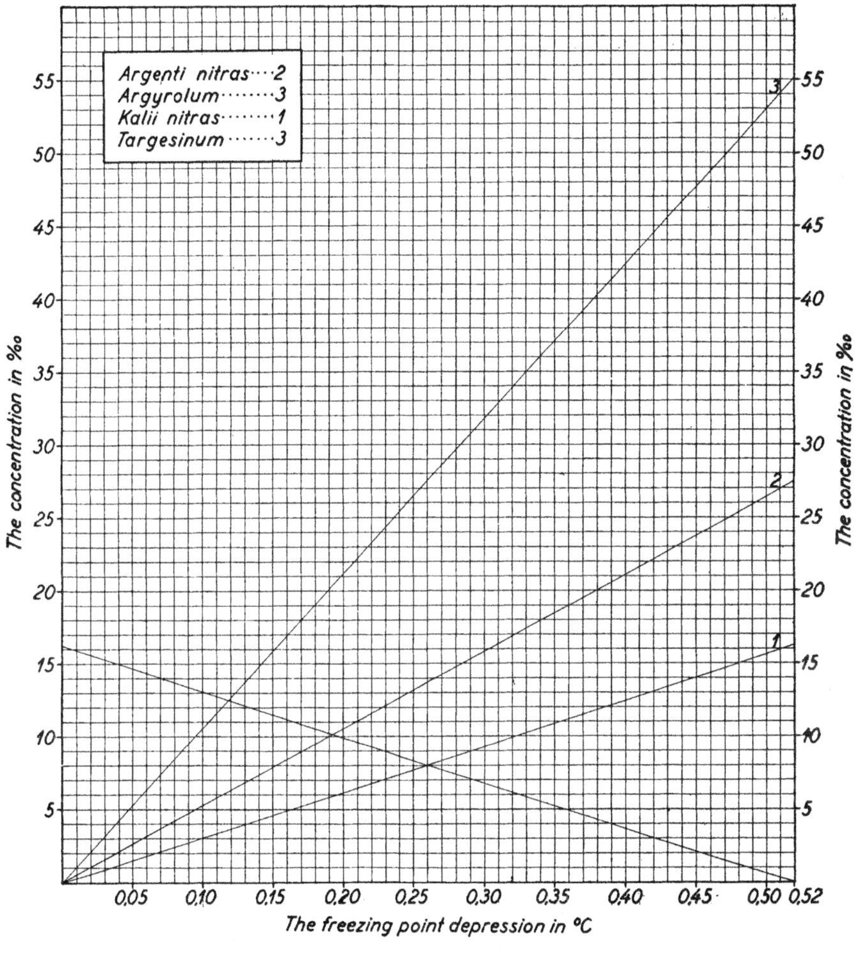
Argenti nitras····2
Argyrolum·········3
Kalii nitras·········1
Targesinum·······3
The concentration in ‰
The concentration in ‰
The freezing point depression in °C
0,05 0,10 0,15 0,20 0,25 0,30 0,35 0,40 0,45 0,50 0,52
5 10 15 20 25 30 35 40 45 50 55
1
2
3

10. References.

1. *Baldes, E. J.:* A Micromethod of Measuring Osmotic Pressure. Journal of Scientific Instruments *11*, 223, 1934.
2. *Bijleveld, J. P. & Dekking, H. M.:* Pijnlooze Oogdruppels. Pharmaceutisch Weekblad *78*, 1229, 1941.
3. *Blegen, E. M.:* Vanndiuresen. Bergen 1940.
4. *Borgen, K. A.:* Lidt om vandsugende Stoffer og Vands Fordampningshastighed. Dansk Tidsskrift for Farmaci 7, 61, 1933.
5. *Bossalino, G.:* Die Geschwindigkeit der Resorption einer Pilocarpinchlorhydratlösung in Abhängigkeit vom osmotischen Druck. Cit. Jahresbericht der Pharmazie *73*, 276, 1938.
6. British Pharmaceutical Codex. London 1934.
7. *Büchi, J. & Baeschlin, E.:* Beitrag zur Herstellung von Augentropfen. Pharm. Acta Helvet. *11*, 103, 1936.
8. *Böhme, H.:* Die Herstellung isotonischer Lösungen. Archiv der Pharmazie *274*, 255, 1936.
9. *Clark, W. M.:* The Determination of Hydrogen Ions. Baltimore 1928.
10. Dispensatorium Danicum. København 1938.
11. *Faurholt, C.:* Almen Kemi og uorganisk Kemi. 4. Udgave. København 1940—41.
12. *Fisher, R. H. & Yates, F.:* Statistical Tables for Biological, Agricultural and Medical Research. London 1938.
13. *Hamburger, M. H. J.:* Méthode pour evaluer la préssion osmotique de trés petites quantités de liquides. Comptes rendus de la société de biologie I, 60, 77, 1906.
14. *Heilbrunn, L. V.:* An Outline of General Physiology. Philadelphia & London 1937.
15. *Henrioul:* Les collyres en pharmacie. Journal de Pharmacie, Belg. *18*, 775, 1936.
16. *Hill, A. V.:* Thermal Method of Measuring the Vapour Pressure of an Aqueous Solution. Proc. Roy. Soc. London Ser. A. *127*, 9, 1930.
17. *Hosford, G. N. & Hicks, A. M.:* Hydrogen Ion Concentration of Tears. Archives of Ophthalmology *13*, 14, 1935.
18. *Jermstad, A.:* Øiendråper og Øienvann. En Oversikt. Norsk Farmaceutisk Tidsskrift 1937.
19. *Jørgensen,* H.: Die Bestimmung der Wasserstoffionenkoncentration. Dresden & Leipzig 1935.

20. *Krogh, A., Lund, C. G. & Pedersen-Bjergaard, K.:* The Osmotic Concentration of Human Lacrymal Fluid. Acta Physiologica Scandinavica *10*, 88, 1945.

21. *Landolt-Börnstein:* Physikalisch-chemische Tabellen, 5. Auflage, Berlin 1923. 5. Auflage, 1 Ergzbd., Berlin 1927. 5. Auflage, 2 Ergzbd., Berlin 1931. 5. Auflage, 3 Ergzbd., Berlin 1936.

22. *Lannung, A.:* Dampfdruckmessungen wässeriger Lösungen der Alkalihalogenide. Zeitschrift für physikalische Chemie A *170*, 134, 1934.

23. — Dampfdruckmessungen des System Calciumchlorid-Wasser. Det kongelige danske Videnskabernes Selsk. Matematisk-fysisk Meddel. *17*, 10, 1940.

24. *Massart, J.:* Sensibilité et adaptation des organismes á la concentration des solutions salines. Arch. d. Biol. *9*, 515, 1889.

25. *Oguchi, C.:* Über den osmotischen Druck der Augentropfen. Arch. f. Ophthalmol. *108*, 363, 1922.

26. *Oguchi, C. & Nakashima, M.:* Über die H-Ionenkoncentrationen der Augensekrete und der Augentropfen. Arch. f. Ophthalmol. *119*, 300, 1927.

27. *Ostwald-Luther:* Physiko-Chemische Messungen. Leipzig 1925.

28. Pharmaconomia Svecica, II, 1944.

29. Pharmacopoea Helvetica, Bern 1933.

30. Remington's Practice of Pharmacy. Philadelphia & London 1936.

31. *Robinson, R. A. & Sinclair, D. A.:* The Activity Coefficients of the Alkali Chlorides and of Lithium Jodide in Aqueous Solution from Vapour Pressure Measurements. Jour. Amer. Chem. Society. *56*, 1830, 1934.

32. *Rosenthaler, L.:* Zur Darstellung isotonischer Lösungen. Schweiz. Apotheker Zt. *78*, 85, 1940.

33. *Roulet, E. L.:* Sur les causes des sensibilité á l'instillation des collyres. Annales d'Oculistique *160*, 241, 1923.

34. *Roth, W. A.:* Physikalisch-chemische Übungen. Leipzig 1916.

35. *v. Röth, A.:* Über die Tränenflüssigkeit. Klinische Monatsbl. f. Augenheilkunde *68*, 598, 1922.

36. *Schou, S. A.:* Dansk Farmaceutisk Aarbog. København 1936.

37. *Sollmann, T.:* A Manual of Pharmacology. Philadelphia & London 1937.

38. *Warburg, E.:* The Osmotic Coefficients of Various Aqueous Solutions of Binary, Ternary, Quaternary and Quinary Sodium and Potassium Salts. Compt. rend. du Lab. Carlsberg, Sér. chim. 22, 547, 1937.

IV. THE PREPARATION OF ISOOSMOTIC SOLUTIONS FOR INJECTION AND FOR LOCAL TREATMENT OF TISSUES

1. Previous investigations of the osmotic pressure of blood.

In preparing solutions that are isoosmotic with blood we have in this treatise primarily considered solutions for parenteral injection as well as such solutions that are used locally in the treatment of injured tissue, and which contain substances as chloramine, euflavine, phenol, hypochlorite, potassium permanganate, and silver nitrate. The aim of our work has been to find experimentally the osmotic pressure that the more frequently applied substances exercise in the more commonly employed concentrations, and on the basis of these determinations a method has been put forward with which isoosmosis can be obtained in extemporaneous prescriptions of hypoosmotic solutions of the said substances. If the solution in question is either isoosmotic or hyperosmotic, an extra addition of sodium chloride, for instance, must, of course, be avoided.

Even if human blood is generally supposed to show a very constant osmotic pressure, a review of the literature concerning this question shows, however, that there are considerable differences between the statements of various authors.

Ascertained by means of *freezing point determinations Dreser* (1892), *Hamburger* (1893), *Winter* (1896) and *v. Koranyi* (1897), all find that blood possesses a freezing point depression of 0.56° C. *Veit* (1900) in normal people finds an average of 0.551°, with variations from 0.501° to 0.605°. *Viola* (1901) in 8 people finds an average of 0.562° with variations from 0.544° to 0.57°. *Krönig & Fueth* (1901) find an average of 0.507°, with variations from 0.490° to 0.509°. *Stewart* (1899) states the freezing point depression of hirudinized blood to be 0.628°, and *Collip* (1920) for defibrinated blood gives values varying from 0.555° to 0.586°.

Ascertained by means of the *hæmatocrit-method* (which is based on the change that takes place in the volume of the red corpuscles when placed in solutions of sodium chloride of different concentrations, as it is taken for granted that the osmotic pressure must be the same in blood as in the solution of sodium chloride in which the corpuscles show the same volume) *Eykman* (1897) finds values corresponding to a freezing point depression varying from 0.537° to 0.568°, the average for 14 determinations being 0.546°. By the same method *Koeppe* (1896) found values from 0.546° to 0.570°, and in the same individual he found variations from day to day of between 0.513° and 0.615°.

Ascertained by means of *vapour pressure determinations* after *Hill*'s (1930) thermo-electric method *Margaria* (1930) in blood of 19 men finds an average value corresponding to a 0.936 % solution of sodium chloride, and in 16 women an average value corresponding to a 0.918 % solution of sodium chloride. These values refer to determinations carried out in an atmosphere of oxygen containing 5 % of carbon dioxide, so that the air in the experimental room had almost the same partial carbon dioxide pressure as has the arterial blood. When, however, the determinations were carried out in an atmosphere of ordinary air the contents of carbon dioxide partly escaped, and now somewhat lower values were found, corresponding to a 0.884 % solution of sodium chloride. By the same method, but employed in the modification described by *Baldes* (1934), *Blegen* (1940) in an extensive trial finds that the osmotic pressure of blood corresponds very nearly with a 0.90 % solution of sodium chloride, and it may be added that *Blegen* has checked the results of the vapour pressure determinations through direct determinations of the osmotic pressure by means of collodion membranes mounted on capillary tubes. *Blegen* found good agreement between the results obtained by the two methods of determination. Finally, we ourselves as a starting point of our investigations, and at the same time as a control of our technique of determination, have taken blood-samples of 10 cubic centimetres from 10 normal men and 10 normal women. The serum, which was centrifuged from the 20 samples of blood, was mixed together, and by the method that we have for the greater part used in this work (*Hill*'s thermo-electric method) showed exactly the same vapour pressure as a 0.9 % solution of sodium chloride. So in this work we have relied on the prevalent view that the osmotic pressure of blood corresponds to a 0.9 % solution of sodium chloride.

As to the technique in using *Hill's* method of determination, applied by us in the modification described by *Baldes* (1934), we refer to the above mentioned statement p. 21—23.

2. Substances examined.

In this work we have included most of the substances that are used in making sterile solutions for injection contained in the Danish pharmacopoeia and the Danish dispensatory, with a few other substances sometimes used in injection therapy. Furthermore we have included some substances, and a few strongly hypotonic solutions that are used locally for the treatment of injured tissue.

We have used highly purified substances for analysis when it has been possible to procure them, otherwise we have employed substances of a purity answering the requirements of the pharmacopoeia.

In order to become acquainted with the concentrations of substances of which it would be expedient to make the determinations, we made a number of calculations, the results of which are given in table 51. The calculations have been made by putting in the respective values in the equation:

$$t = \frac{n \cdot k \cdot g \cdot 1000}{M \cdot L}$$

t being the freezing point depression that the solution shows in relation to the solvent, n being the number of ions into which the substance is dissociated, k being the molar freezing point depression of the solvent, g the weight of the dissolved substance in grammes, M the molecular weight of the dissolved substance, and L the total volume of substance and solvent.

Off the substances shown in table 51 is noted, where possible, the number of ions, n, into which the substances are probably dissociated, the molecular weights, and the concentrations, (expressed in grammes in 1000 millilitres), that should be expected to give a freezing point depression of 0.20°, 0.40°, 0.56°, and 0.80° respectively, calculated after the above mentioned equation.

Figures 17, 18, 19, and 20 have been drawn on the basis of the values in table 51. The concentration, expressed in grammes in a solution of 1000 millilitres, has been chosen for ordinate, and the freezing point depression, expressed in °C, for abscissa.

Table 51.

A list of the 67 substances included in the investigations in this part of the work.

n	M.	0.20°	0.40°	0.56°	0.80°	A graphical representation of: I The values calculated according to Raoult's law	II A comparison between the calculated and the experimentally found values	III The values found experimentally and for practical use shown together with the mirrored NaCl curve
						shown in figure:		
1 Acid. ascorbinicum ..	176.06	18.93	37.85	53.01	75.71	17	23	34
1 Acid. boricum	61.84	6.65	13.30	18.62	26.60	19	22	38
1 Acid. citricum	210.08	22.58	45.17	63.26	90.33	20	24	33
1 Acid. nicotinicum....	123.05	13.23	26.46	37.05	52.91	20	27	36
1 Aethylendiamini hydras	78.10	8.40	16.79	23.52	33.58	20	29	36
1 Alcohol absolutus ..	46.05	4.95	9.90	13.87	19.80	19		23
3 Amphetamini sulfas.	368.30	13.20	26.41	36.97	52.81	18	26	33
2 Aneurini hydrochlor.	337.17	18.12	36.25	50.76	72.49	18	23	34
1 Antipyrinum	188.12	20.22	40.45	56.64	80.89	18	21	31
2 Apomorphini hydrchl.	312.61	16.80	33.61	47.06	67.21	20	28	37
1 Arseni trioxydum ..	197.86	21.27	42.54	59.58	85.08	20	29	33
3 Calcii chloridum	219.10	7.85	15.70	21.99	31.40	19	28	37
3 Calcii gluconas	448.27	16.06	32.13	44.99	64.25	17	27	36
2 Chinini hydrochlorid.	396.71	21.32	42.65	59.72	85.29	18	27	36
Chiniophonum							22	38
Chloraminum	281.63						25	38
2 Cincaini hydrochlor.	379.91	20.42	40.84	57.20	81.68	17	26	39
2 Codeini hydrochlorid.	371.68	19.98	39.96	55.96	79.91	18	28	37
2 Codeini phosphas....	424.25	22.80	45.61	63.87	91.21	19	21	31
2 Diemalnatrium	206.10	11.08	22.16	31.03	44.31	20	28	37
2 Emetini hydrochlorid.	553.28	29.74	59.48	83.30	118.96	20	23	34
2 Ephedrini hydrochlor.	201.60	10.84	21.68	30.35	43.35	17	27	36
Euflavinum							29	38
3 Ferrosi lactas	287.97	10.32	20.64	28.90	41.28	18	27	36
1 Glucosum (anhydricum)	180.10	19.36	38.72	54.23	77.44	19	22	33
1 Glycerinum	92.06	9.90	19.79	27.72	39.59	19	27	36
1 Hexamethylentetram.	140.13	15.06	30.13	42.19	60.26	19	29	32
3 Jodphtaleinum	865.78	31.02	62.05	86.90	124.10	19	25	35
2 Kalii chloridum	74.56	4.01	8.02	11.23	16.03	17	28	36
2 Kalii jodidum	166.03	8.92	17.85	25.00	35.70	17	21	36
2 Kalii permanganas ..	158.03	8.49	16.98	23.78	33.97	17	29	38
2 Kalii phosphas KH_2PO_4	136.14	7.32	14.64	20.50	29.27	17	28	39
2 Lobelini hydrochlor...	373.69	20.09	40.17	56.26	80.34	17	27	36
2 Magnii sulfas	246.49	13.25	26.50	37.11	53.00	19	23	34
3 Mercuranum	750.51	26.90	53.80	75.40	107.60	20	25	38
2 Mersalylum	505.79	27.20	54.40	76.14	108.80	17	24	32
2 Morphini hydrochlor.	375.68	20.19	40.39	56.56	80.77	19	29	33
2 Narcotini hydrochlor.	467.68	25.14	50.28	70.41	100.55	18	24	32

n		M.	0.20°	0.40°	0.56°	0.80°	A graphical representation of I The values calculated according to Raoult's law	II A comparison between the calculated and the experimentally found values	III The values found experimentally, and for practical use shown together with the mirrored NaCl curve
							shown in figure:		
3	Natrii arsenas $Na_2HAsO_4 \cdot 7H_2O$	312.05	11.18	22.36	31.32	44.73	19	25	33
2	Natrii benzoas	144.04	7.74	15.48	21.69	30.97	20	23	39
2	Natrii bicarbonas	84.01	4.52	9.03	12.65	18.06	20	27	36
4	Natrii citras $C_6H_5O_7Na_3 \cdot 2H_2O$	294.07	7.90	15.81	22.14	31.61	18	27	36
2	Natrii jodidum	149.93	8.06	16.12	22.57	32.23	17	25	36
2	Natrii nitris	69.01	3.71	7.42	10.39	14.88	19	22	37
3	Natrii phosphas	268.14	9.61	19.22	26.97	38.44	18	26	35
3	Natrii phosphas $Na_2HPO_4, 2H_2O$	178.06	6.38	12.76	17.87	25.53	18	28	37
2	Natrii salicylas	160.04	8.60	17.20	24.09	34.41	19	24	35
3	Natrii sulfas	322.22	11.55	23.09	32.34	46.18	18	21	35
3	Natrii thiosulfas	248.20	8.89	17.79	24.91	35.58	18	26	34
1	Nicaethamidum	178.13	19.15	38.30	53.63	76.60	20	25	32
1	Nicotinamidum	122.07	13.12	26.25	36.76	52.49	17	21	32
3	Oxedrini tartras	484.28	17.35	34.71	48.57	69.41	19	22	31
	Oxychinolini sulfas							24	38
2	Oxyconi hydrochlorid.	405.69	21.81	43.62	61.10	87.24	18	22	39
2	Papaverini hydrochlor.	375.65	20.19	40.38	56.55	80.76	20	27	36
	Pentazolum	138.12	14.85	29.70	41.59	59.39	20	24	31
2	Phenemalnatrium	254.11	13.66	27.32	38.26	54.63	18	22	31
1	Phenolum	94.05	10.11	22.23	28.31	40.45	20	29	38
	Phenosalylum							29	38
2	Procaini hydrochlorid.	272.65	14.65	29.31	41.05	58.62	17	26	35
1	Saccharum	342.18	36.78	73.57	103.03	147.14	18	21	31
1	Saccharum lactis	360.19	38.74	77.47	108.40	154.90	17	21	34
2	Strychnini nitras	397.21	21.35	42.70	59.80	85.40	17	29	37
	Tanninum							25	38
2	Tetracaini hydrochlr.	286.61	15.42	30.83	43.18	61.66	18	26	39
1	Theophyllinum	198.12	21.30	42.60	59.65	85.19	19	28	36
1	Urethanum	89.07	9.58	19.15	26.82	38.30	20	28	37

In many previous proposals for the preparation of isotonic solutions the authors have only worked with the calculated values shown in the above table 51 and figures 17—20. That these values in certain cases may differ rather widely from the actual osmotic conditions will appear from the sequel, where we are giving a more detailed account of the values we have found through experimental determinations, which are shown in tables 52—142. In figures 21—

Fig. 17

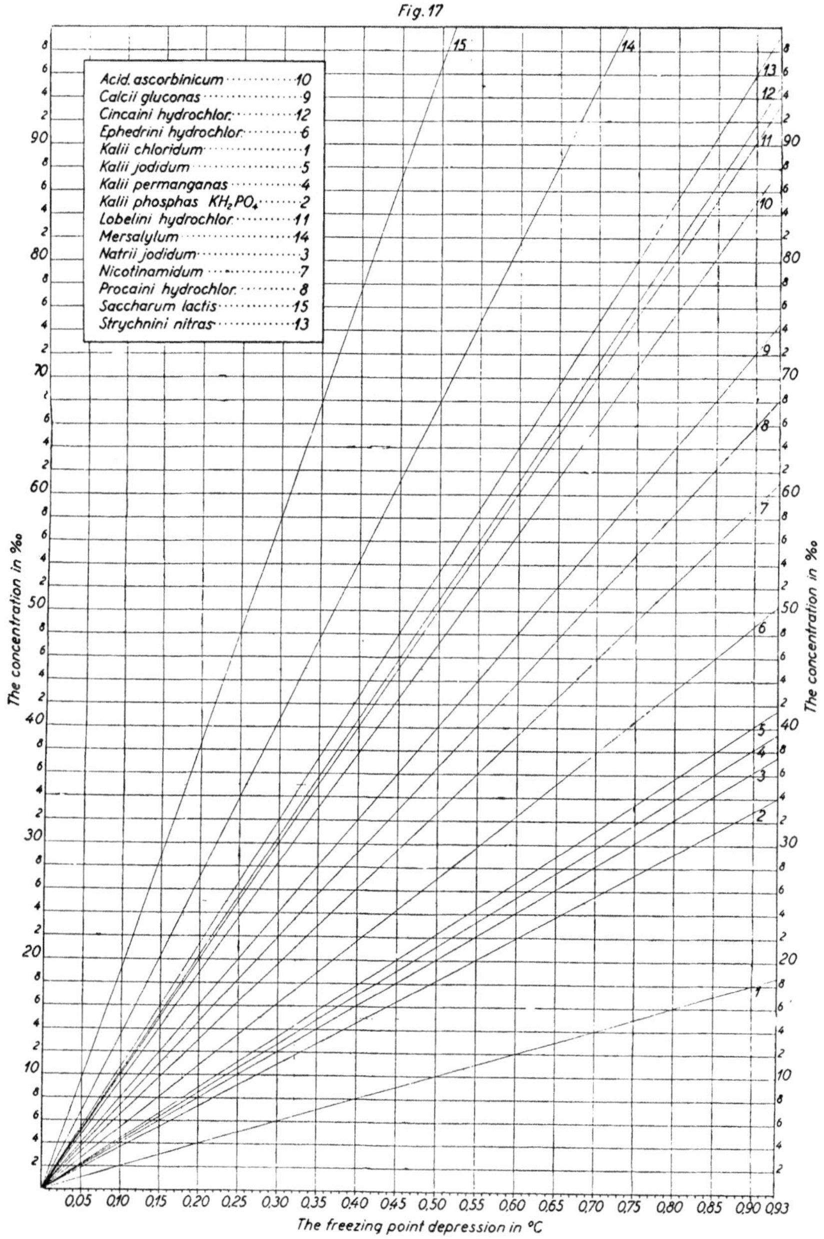
Acid. ascorbinicum 10
Calcii gluconas 9
Cincaini hydrochlor. 12
Ephedrini hydrochlor. 6
Kalii chloridum 1
Kalii jodidum 5
Kalii permanganas 4
Kalii phosphas KH_2PO_4 2
Lobelini hydrochlor. 11
Mersalylum 14
Natrii jodidum 3
Nicotinamidum 7
Procaini hydrochlor. 8
Saccharum lactis 15
Strychnini nitras 13
The concentration in ‰
The freezing point depression in °C
0,05 0,10 0,15 0,20 0,25 0,30 0,35 0,40 0,45 0,50 0,55 0,60 0,65 0,70 0,75 0,80 0,85 0,90 0,93

Fig. 18

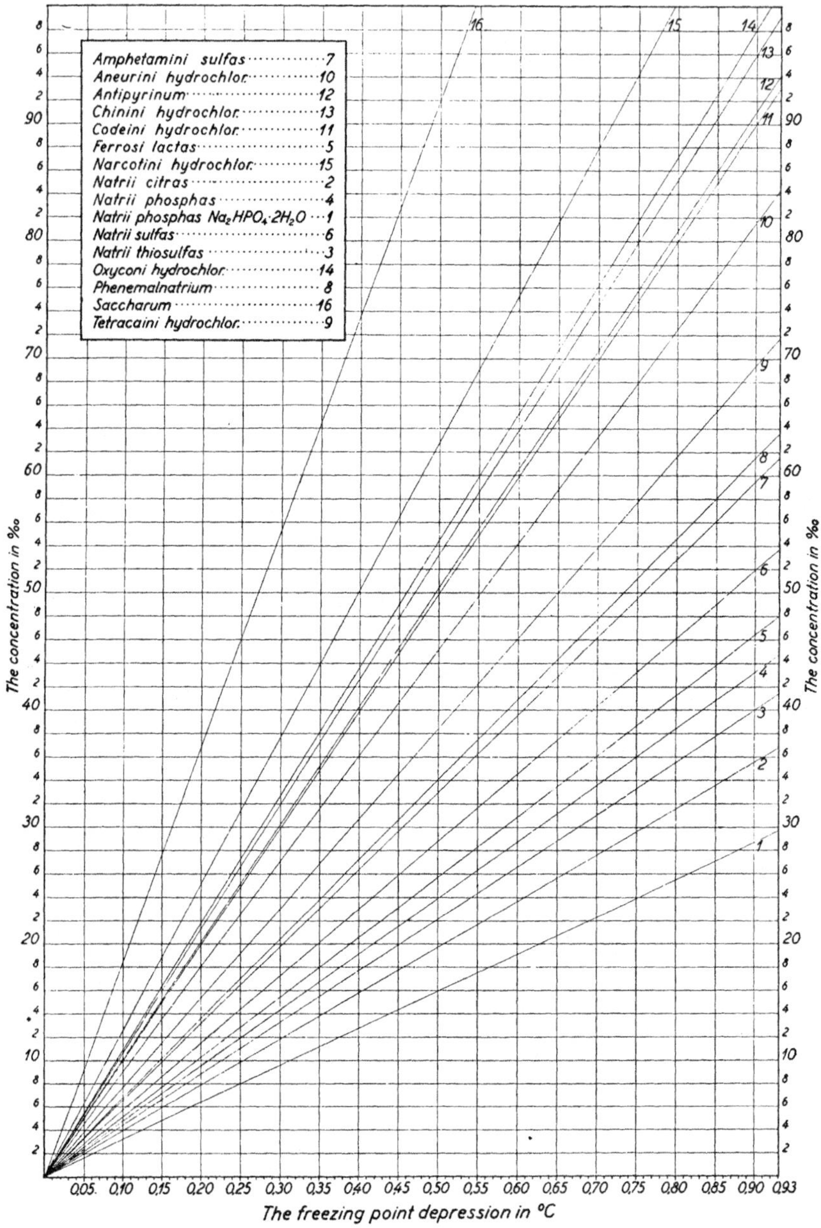

Amphetamini sulfas 7
Aneurini hydrochlor. 10
Antipyrinum 12
Chinini hydrochlor. 13
Codeini hydrochlor. 11
Ferrosi lactas 5
Narcotini hydrochlor. 15
Natrii citras 2
Natrii phosphas 4
Natrii phosphas $Na_2HPO_4 \cdot 2H_2O$ ... 1
Natrii sulfas 6
Natrii thiosulfas 3
Oxyconi hydrochlor. 14
Phenemalnatrium 8
Saccharum 16
Tetracaini hydrochlor. 9
The concentration in ‰
The freezing point depression in °C
0,05 0,10 0,15 0,20 0,25 0,30 0,35 0,40 0,45 0,50 0,55 0,60 0,65 0,70 0,75 0,80 0,85 0,90 0,93
10 20 30 40 50 60 70 80 90

Fig. 19

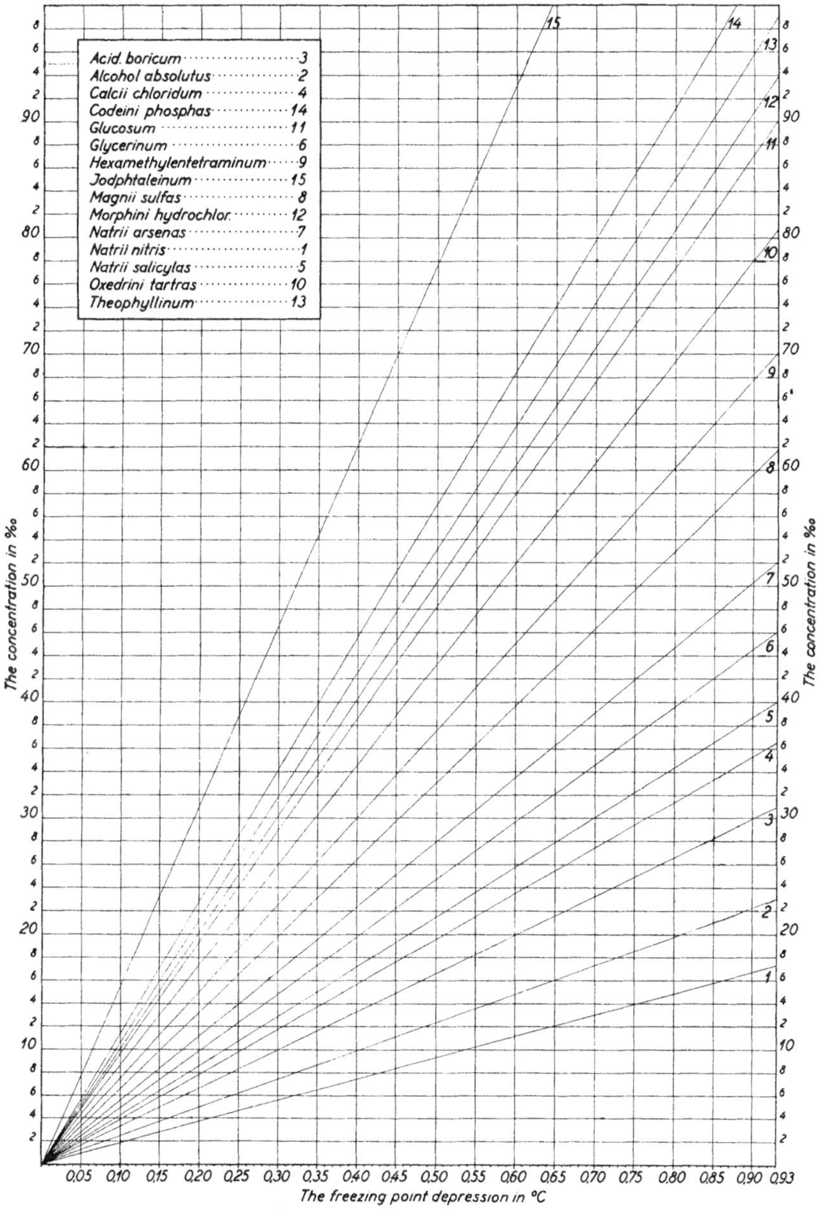
Acid. boricum 3
Alcohol absolutus 2
Calcii chloridum 4
Codeini phosphas 14
Glucosum 11
Glycerinum 6
Hexamethylentetraminum 9
Jodphtaleinum 15
Magnii sulfas 8
Morphini hydrochlor. 12
Natrii arsenas 7
Natrii nitris 1
Natrii salicylas 5
Oxedrini tartras 10
Theophyllinum 13
The concentration in ‰
The freezing point depression in °C

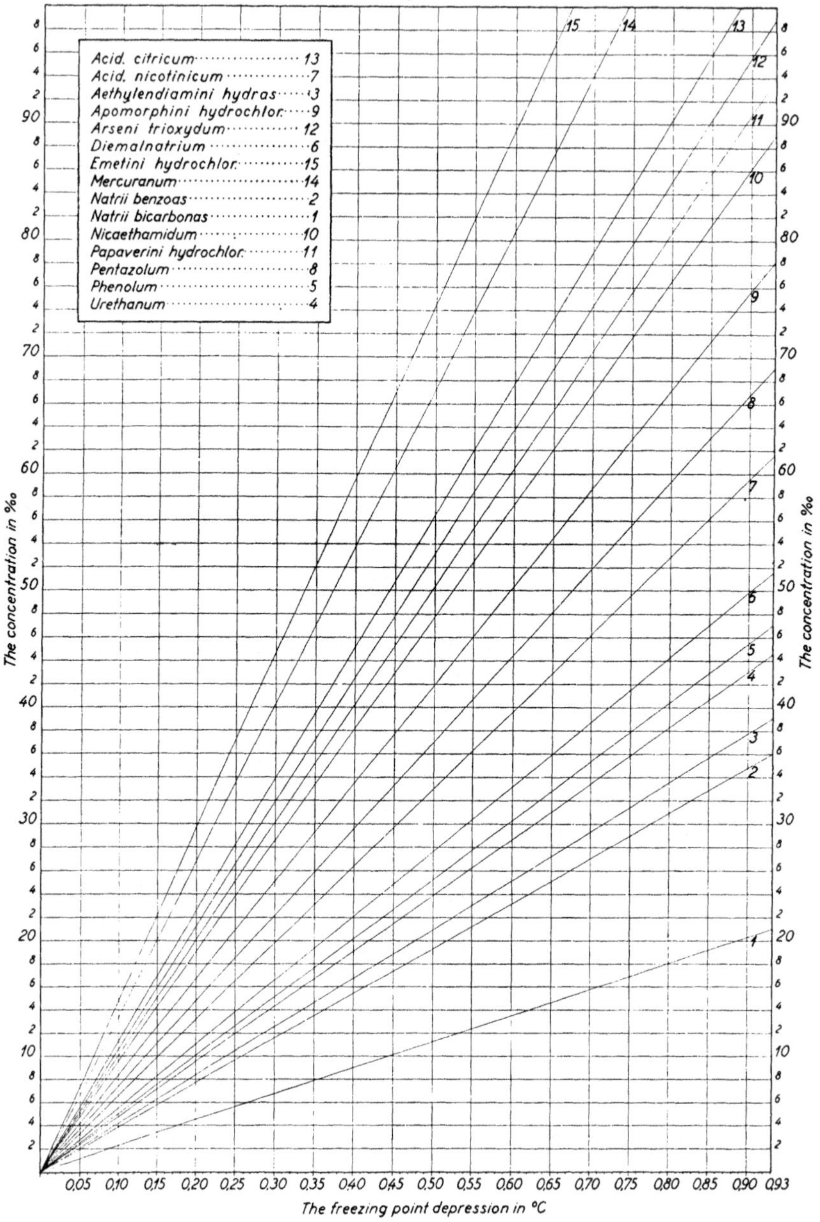

Acid. citricum 13
Acid. nicotinicum 7
Aethylendiamini hydras 3
Apomorphini hydrochlor. 9
Arseni trioxydum 12
Diemalnatrium 6
Emetini hydrochlor. 15
Mercuranum 14
Natrii benzoas 2
Natrii bicarbonas 1
Nicaethamidum 10
Papaverini hydrochlor. 11
Pentazolum 8
Phenolum 5
Urethanum 4
The concentration in ‰
The freezing point depression in °C
0,05 0,10 0,15 0,20 0,25 0,30 0,35 0,40 0,45 0,50 0,55 0,60 0,65 0,70 0,75 0,80 0,85 0,90 0,93

Fig. 20

29 both the calculated and the experimentally found values have been marked in pairs, so that the reader should be able quickly to estimate the difference between the theoretically calculated and the values actually found.

The results found have been given in the tables 52—142, each of the substances in its own table. The substances have not been given in alphabetical order, but according to the succession in which they enter the accompanying figures. In far the greater number of cases the results have been arrived at by a determination of the vapour pressure, from which the corresponding freezing point depression has then been calculated. In a few cases, where it has been possible to obtain reliable vapour pressure determinations, the freezing point depression has been determined by means of *Beckmann*'s thermometer.

In the case of two substances, determinations of both vapour pressure and freezing point depression have been made of the same solutions, to show how great an agreement can be obtained with these two methods of determination. Where results are to be found in the literature of other authors, we have in the case of each single substance made a comparison between the results found by others, and those obtained by us.

3. *Results.*

Antipyrinum.

Vapour pressure determinations were made of the following solutions of phenazone. In table 52 the results have been given in the corresponding freezing point depressions.

Table 52.

The concentration of phenazone grammes / 1000 millilitres	7.50	15.00	30.00	45.00	60.00	90.00
The corresponding freezing point depression in °C	0.71	0.134	0.246	0.368	0.473	0.656

The values given in table 52 are in good agreement with the values given by *Schou:* that a 1 % solution of phenazone corresponds to a 0.15 % solution of sodium chloride, which gives a freezing point depression of 0.091°, while we, according to fig. 21, arrive at 0.094°. *Rosenthaler*'s value, however, of 0.80° for an 8.1 % solution of phenazone, differs considerably from our results, as we find that an 11 % solution of phenazone gives a freezing point depression of 0.80°. On the other hand, *Rosenthaler*'s value agrees precisely with the value calculated by us (given in table 51), which goes to show that the values given in literature must be taken with great reservation, these figures often referring to simply calculated values with no consideration to the activity of the substances.

Codeini phosphas.

Vapour pressure determinations were made of the following solutions of codeine phosphate. In table 53 the results have been given in the corresponding freezing point depressions.

Table 53.

The concentration of codeine phosphate grammes / 1000 millilitres	7.50	15.00	30.00	45.00	60.00	90.00
The corresponding freezing point depression in °C.	0.059	0.115	0.223	0.329	0.430	0.615

We have found no values in literature with which to compare our values for this substance.

Kalii jodidum.

Vapour pressure determinations were made of the following solutions of potassium iodide. In table 54 the results have been given in the corresponding freezing point depressions.

Table 54.

The concentration of potassium iodide grammes / 1000 millilitres	5.00	10.00	20.00	40.00
The corresponding freezing point depression in °C.	0.104	0.207	0.401	0.795

In table 55 the values for potassium iodide of other authors are compared with our own values.

Table 55.

Author	The concentration in %	The freezing point depression	The freezing point depression found by us according to fig. 21
Landolt-Börnstein 1923	0.300	0.0637	0.063
» »	1.500	0.308	0.305
» »	3.083	0.626	0.613
Böhme	0.46	0.10	0.096
»	0.94	0.20	0.193
»	1.96	0.40	0.394
»	3.96	0.80	0.786
Rosenthaler	2.75	0.56	0.549
Own result	2.59		0.520

In table 55 there is a good agreement between the values which other authors have given for potassium iodide, and the values found by us.

Natrii sulfas.

Vapour pressure determinations were made of the following solutions of sodium sulphate. The results, changed into the corresponding freezing point depressions, are shown in table 56.

Table 56.

The concentration of Na_2SO_4 grammes/ 1000 millilitres	7.50	15.00	25.00	30.00	45.00	50.00	60.00	70.00
The corresponding freezing point depression in ^{0}C.	0.112	0.215	0.325	0.409	0.588	0.636	0.759	0.881

In table 57 the sodium sulphate values of other authors are compared with our own values.

Table 57.

Author	The concentration in $^0/_0$	The freezing point depression	The freezing point depression found by us according to fig. 21
Landolt-Börnstein 1923	1.6125	0.2297	0.230
»	3.225	0.4340	0.433
»	6.450	0.8141	0.816
Landolt-Börnstein 1931	0.7965	0.1134	0.120
»	1.618	0.2183	0.230
»	3.215	0.4056	0.432
Remington	1.0	0.15	0.148
»	4.07	0.56	0.536
Own result	3.95		0.520
Brit. Pharm. Codex 1934 and Ph. Helvet.	1.0	0.15	0.148
Rosenthaler	4.20	0.56	0.648

In table 57 it will be seen that there is a good agreement between *Landolt-Börnstein*'s values from 1923, and ours. On the other hand, the agreement is not so good with the *Landolt-Börnstein* values from 1931, the latter being about 5 % lower. This disagreement is evidently due to the fact that the two different years of the *L—B* tables refer to two different sources. It will be seen that there is a good agreement between *Remington*'s, *Ph. Helwet.*'s, and our values, whereas *Rosenthaler*'s value somewhat disagrees with ours. The concentration that is isoosmotic with blood amounts to about 4 % (*Remington:* 4.07 %, *Rosenthaler:* 4.20 %, *we:* 3.95 %).

Nicotinamidum.

Vapour pressure determinations were made of the following solutions of nicotinamide. In table 58 the results are given in the corresponding freezing point depressions.

Table 58.

The concentration af nicotinamide grammes / 1000 millilitres	7.50	15.00	30.00	45.00	60.00	80.00
The corresponding freezing point depression in °C.	0.116	0.206	0.375	0.518	0.661	0.842

We have found no values in literature with which to compare our results.

Saccharum.

Vapour pressure determinations were made of the following solutions of sucrose. In table 59 the results are given in the corresponding freezing point depressions.

Table 59.

The concentration of sucrose grammes/1000 millilitres	7.50	15.00	30.00	45.00	60.00	90.00	120.0
The corresponding freezing point depression in °C.	0.033	0.073	0.151	0.239	0.333	0.493	0.692

In table 60 a comparison has been made between the sucrose values of other authors, and our own values.

Table 60.

Author	The concentration in %	The freezing point depression	The freezing point depression found by us according to fig. 21
Brit. Pharm. Codex 1934	1.0	0.054	0.047
Landolt-Börnstein 1923	0.6878	0.0378	0.031
» »	3.596	0.1963	0.188
» »	9.718	0.5387	0.550
Ph. Helvet. and Remington ..	1.0	0.054	0.047
» ..	10.0	0.56	0.567
Böhme	10.3	0.56	0.585
Schou	10.0	0.56	0.567
Rosenthaler	10.0	0.56	0.567
Own result	9.25		0.520

As to the agreement between the values for sucrose found by others, and those found by us, a great difference is seen in table 60 in the case of the weaker concentrations, *Landolt-Börnstein* in a solution of approximately 0.7 %, and *Brit. Pharm. Codex, Ph. Helvet.*, and *Remington* in a 1 % solution finding freezing point depressions about 15 to 20 % greater than those found by us. The concentration that is isoosmotic with blood is stated to be 10 % by *Ph. Helvet., Remington, Böhme, Schou,* and *Rosenthaler*. All the authors evidently have calculated this value from the supposition that the system is ideal, so that the calculated and the experimentally found values should coincide. We find experimentally, however, that the isoosmotic concentration is 9.25 %.

Saccharum lactis.

Vapour pressure determinations were made of the following solutions of lactose. In table 61 the results are given in the corresponding freezing point depressions.

Table 61.

The concentration of lactose grammes / 1000 millilitres ..	7.50	15.00	30.00	60.00	90.00	120.0
The corresponding freezing point depression in °C.	0.028	0.066	0.146	0.296	0.471	0.656

In table 62 a comparison has been made between the lactose values of other authors, and our own values.

Table 62.

Author	The concentration in %	The freezing point depression	The freezing point depression found by us according to fig. 21
Landolt-Börnstein 1936	4.988	0.280	0.246
»	9.949	0.557	0.532
Ph. Helvet.	1.0	0.07	0.040
»	9.4	0.56	0.498
Remington	1.0	0.07	0.040
»	9.4	0.56	0.498
Rosenthaler	9.50	0.56	0.503
Own result	9.75		0.520

The values in *Ph. Helvet.*'s and *Remington*'s tables are identical, and like the values in *Landolt-Börnstein*'s tables somewhat greater than ours, especially in the case of the weaker concentration. The concentration that is isoosmotic with blood is stated to be 9.4 % by *Ph. Helv.* and *Remington,* and 9.5 % by *Rosenthaler.* We find 9.75 %, and *Landolt-Börnstein* 9.95 %.

In fig. 21 the values from the tables 52, 53, 54, 56, 58, 59, and 61 have been marked as small circles. The complete curves, made by connecting these circles, have been arrived at in the following manner: in a system of coordinates, where the logarithm of the concentration has been marked along the ordinate, and the logarithm of the freezing point depression along the abscissa, the above mentioned determined values have been marked. It now proved that the curve connecting the marked points practically always formed a straight line. By transferring the straight line of the logarithmic system, point by point, to the arithmetical system used in fig. 21, in most cases we arrive at more or less arched curves. It is evident that on the basis of the limited number of practicable determinations a straight line is much more accurately drawn in the logarithmic system than is a curved line in the arithmetical system. We have chosen the arithmetical system of coordinates, because in the daily work this system is easier to work with, but originally the curves were drawn in the logarithmic system, and, as mentioned, transferred to the other system in order to obtain the greatest possible accuracy. The values in fig. 21 have thus been marked in the same manner as the values in fig. 6.

Fig.21

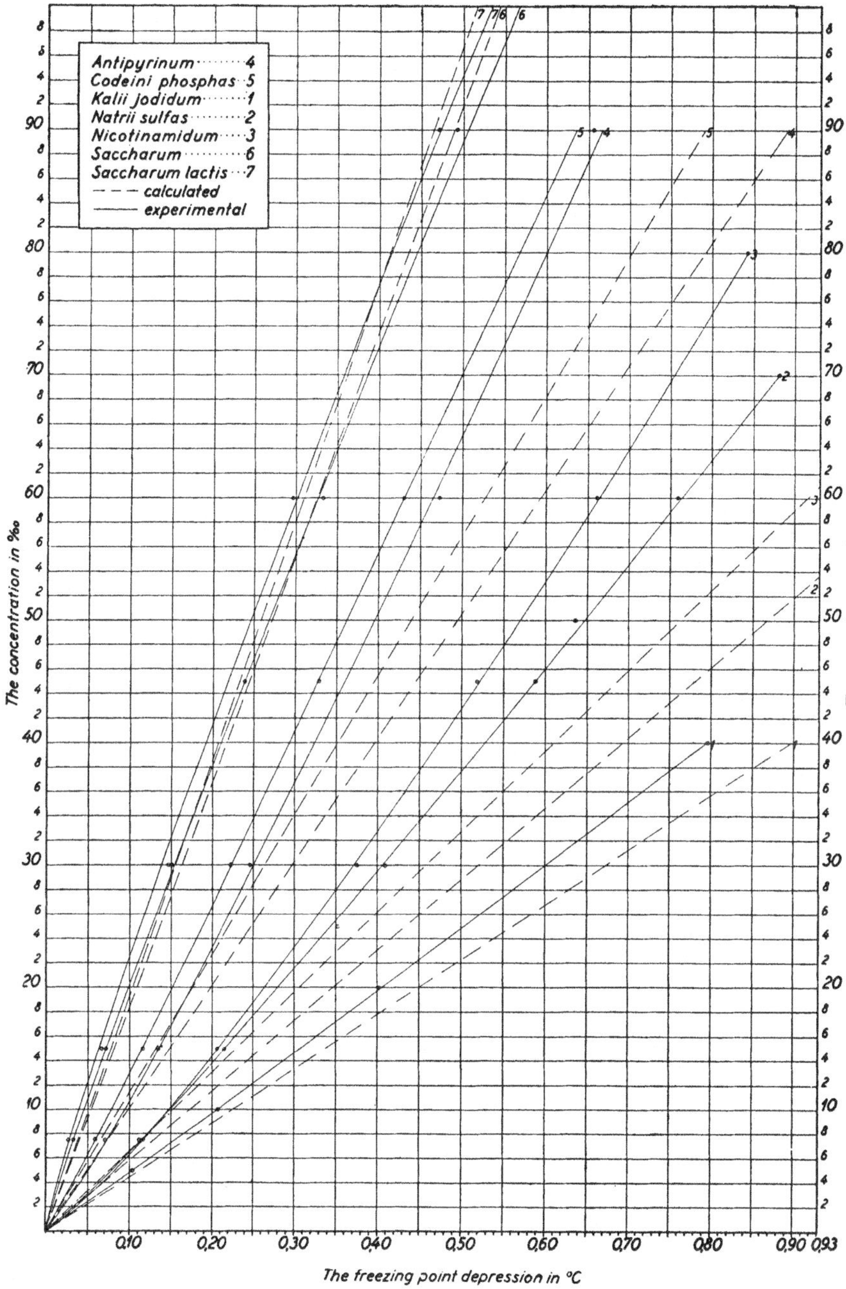
Antipyrinum 4
Codeini phosphas 5
Kalii jodidum 1
Natrii sulfas 2
Nicotinamidum 3
Saccharum 6
Saccharum lactis 7
calculated
experimental
The concentration in ‰
The freezing point depression in °C

Acidum boricum.

Vapour pressure determinations were made of the following solutions of boric acid. In table 63 the results are given in the corresponding freezing point depressions.

Table 63.

The concentration of boric acid grammes / 1000 millilitres	0.333	0.665	1.330	2.660	3.000
The corresponding freezing point depression in °C.	0.100	0.197	0.388	0.676	0.794

In table 64 a comparison has been made between the values for boric acid of other authors and our own values.

Table 64.

Author	The concentration in %	The freezing point depression	The freezing point depression found by us according to fig. 22
Brit. Pharm. Codex 1934	1.0	0.25	0.283
» »	2.2	0.56	0.297
» »	3.1	0.86	0.825
Landolt-Börnstein 1923	0.410	0.129	0.121
» »	1.024	0.318	0.290
» »	1.55	0.489	0.428
Landolt-Börnstein 1931	0.325	0.084	0.097
» »	0.902	0.236	0.257
» »	1.723	0.441	0.474
» »	2.573	0.665	0.693
» »	2.938	0.760	0.786
Ph. Helvet. and Remington ..	1.0	0.25	0.283
» » ..	2.2	0.56	0.597
» » ..	3.1	0.80	0.825
Rosenthaler	2.75	0.80	0.738
Schou	1.0	0.276	0.283
Own result	1.9		0.520

It will be seen from the values of the freezing point depression in table 64, that our figures are lower than *Landolt-Börnstein*'s (1923) and *Rosenthaler*'s, but higher than *Landolt-Börnstein*'s (1931), *Ph. Helvet.'s, Remington*'s and *Schou*'s. The isoosmotic concentration is stated to be 2.2 % by *Ph. Helvet.*, and *Remington*, and we find it to be 1.9 %.

Chiniophonum.

Vapour pressure determinations were made of the following solutions of chiniofon. In table 65 the results are given in the corresponding freezing point depressions.

Table 65.

The concentration of chiniofon grammes/1000 millilitres	5.00	10.00	20.00	30.00
The corresponding freezing point depression in °C.	0.038	0.074	0.144	0.200

We have found no results in literature with which to compare our values.

Glucosum.

Vapour pressure determinations were made of the following solutions of dextrose ($C_6H_{12}O_6$). In table 66 the results are given in the corresponding freezing point depressions.

Table 66.

The concentration of dextrose grammes/ 1000 millilitres	7.82	15.63	25.00	31.25	40.00	50.00	62.50	80.00
The corresponding freezing point depression in °C.	0.078	0.154	0.255	0.318	0.406	0.524	0.646	0.828

In table 67 a comparison has been made between the values for dextrose of other authors, and our own values.

Table 67.

Author	The concentration in %	The freezing point depression	The freezing point depression found by us according to fig. 22
Brit. Pharm. Codex 1934	1.0	0.10	0.100
» »	5.1	0.56	0.526
Landolt-Börnstein 1923	0.3566	0.0363	0.036
» »	0.8464	0.0870	0.085
» »	2.388	0.2475	0.243
» »	7.342	0.7719	0.759
Böhme	5.4	0.56	0.557
Remington and Ph. Helvet.	5.0	0.56	0.515
Rosenthaler	5.10	0.56	0.526
Own result	5.05		0.520

In table 67 there is a good agreement between the values of the various authors. Thus the concentration that is isoosmotic with blood is stated to be 5.0 % by *Ph. Helvet.* and *Remington,* while we find 5.05 %, *Brit. Pharm. Codex* and *Rosenthaler* 5.10 %, and *Böhme* 5.4 %. The latter value, however, is evidently a calculated one.

Natrii nitris.

Vapour pressure determinations were made of the following solutions of sodium nitrite. In table 68 the results are given in the corresponding freezing point depressions.

Table 68.

The concentration of sodium nitrite grammes / 1000 millilitres	5.00	10.00	20.00
The corresponding freezing point depression in °C. ..	0.248	0.481	0.925

We have found no results in literature with which to compare our results.

Oxedrini tartras.

Vapour pressure determinations were made of the following solutions of neo-synephrine tartrate. In table 69 the results are given in the corresponding freezing point depressions.

Table 69.

The concentration of neo-synephrine tartrate grammes / 1000 millilitres	7.50	15.00	30.00	45.00	60.00	90.00
The corresponding freezing point depression in °C.	0.080	0.150	0.282	0.411	0.624	0.762

We have found no values in literature with which to compare our results.

Oxyconi hydrochloridum.

Vapour pressure determinations were made of the following solutions of eukodal. In table 70 the results are given in the corresponding freezing point depressions.

Table 70.

The concentration of eukodal grammes/1000 millilitres	6.25	12.50	25.00	50.00	100.0
The corresponding freezing point depression in °C.	0.052	0.100	0.191	0.367	0.677

We have found no results in literature with which to compare our values.

Phenemalnatrium.

Vapour pressure determinations were made of the following solutions of soluble phenobarbitone. In table 71 the results are given in the corresponding freezing point depressions.

Table 71.

The concentration of soluble phenobarbitone grammes/1000 millilitres ..	7.50	15.00	30.00	45.00	60.00
The corresponding freezing point depression in °C.	0.101	0.201	0.396	0.587	0.778

We have found no values in literature with which to compare our values.

In fig. 22 the values from tables 63, 65, 66, 68, 69, 70, and 71 have been marked in the same manner as the values in fig. 6.

Fig. 22

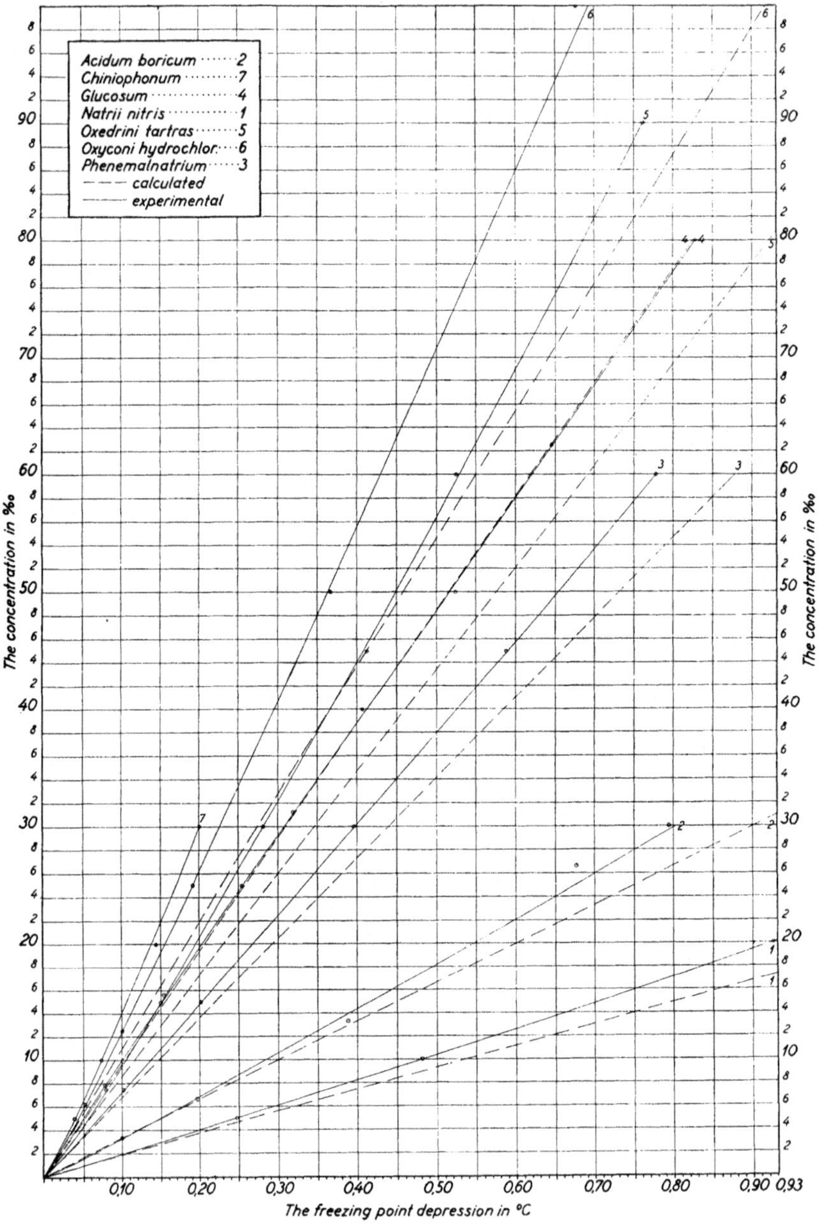
Acidum boricum ······ 2
Chiniophonum ········ 7
Glucosum ············ 4
Natrii nitris ········· 1
Oxedrini tartras ······· 5
Oxyconi hydrochlor. ··· 6
Phenemalnatrium ······ 3
calculated
experimental
The concentration in ‰
The freezing point depression in °C

Acidum ascorbinicum.

Vapour pressure determinations were made of the following solutions of ascorbic acid. In table 72 the results are given in the corresponding freezing point depressions.

Table 72.

The concentration of ascorbic acid grammes/1000 millilitres	7.50	15.00	30.00	60.00	90.00
The corresponding freezing point depression in °C.	0.081	0.157	0.311	0.610	0.923

We have found no values in literature with which to compare our results.

Aneurini hydrochloridum.

Vapour pressure determinations were made of the following solutions of aneurine hydrochloride. In table 73 the results are given in the corresponding freezing point depressions.

Table 73.

The concentration of aneurine hydrochloride grammes/1000 millilitres	7.50	15.00	30.00	45.00	60.00	75.00
The corresponding freezing point depression in °C.	0.108	0.207	0.376	0.543	0.715	0.872

We have found no values in literature with which to compare our results.

Emetini hydrochloridum.

Vapour pressure determinations were made of the following solutions of emetine hydrochloride. In table 74 the results are given in the corresponding freezing point depressions.

Table 74.

The concentration of emetine hydrochloride grammes/1000 millilitres	7.50	15.00	30.00	60.00
The corresponding freezing point depression in °C.	0.045	0.090	0.176	0.324

In table 75 a comparison is made between the emetine hydrochloride values of other authors, and our own.

Table 75.

Author	The concentration in %	The freezing point depression	The freezing point depression found by us according to fig. 23
Schou	1.0	0.056	0.062
Brit. Pharm. Codex 1934, Ph. Helvet., Remington and van Itallie	1.0	0.088	0.062
Ph. Helvet. and Remington	3.0	0.240	0.171
Ph. Helvet., Remington and van Itallie	5.0	0.341	0.274
Rosenthaler	8.00	0.56	0.423
Own result	10.0		0.520

The values in table 75 show that there is an enormous difference between the values of other authors and our own. For instance, in the case of a 1 % solution of emetine hydrochloride, *Schou*'s value is about 10 % lower than ours, whereas *Brit. Pharm. Codex, Ph. Helvet., Remington,* and *van Itallie* give values that are about 40 % higher. The concentration that is isoosmotic with blood is stated by *Rosenthaler* to be 8 %, which almost corresponds to the calculated concentration, whereas we find experimentally that it is 10 %.

Magnii sulfas.

Vapour pressure determinations were made of the following solutions of magnesium sulphate. In table 76 the results are given in the corresponding freezing point depressions.

Table 76.

The concentration of magnesium sulphate grammes/1000 millilitres	7.50	15.00	30.00	45.00	60.00	90.00
The corresponding freezing point depression in °C.	0.070	0.134	0.261	0.374	0.500	0.706

In table 77 a comparison is made between the values for magnesium sulphate of other authors and our own values.

There is a fairly good agreement between the values in table 77. The concentration which is isoosmotic with blood is stated to be

Table 77.

Author	The concentration in %	The freezing point depression	The freezing point depression found by us according to fig. 23
Brit. Pharm. Codex 1934	1.0	0.08	0.094
» »	6.35	0.56	0.523
Landolt-Börnstein 1923	0.7401	0.0742	0.071
» »	2.220	0.2035	0.196
» »	4.939	0.4158	0.413
Ph. Helvet. and Remington ..	1.0	0.08	0.094
» » ..	6.6	0.56	0.543
Rosenthaler	6.60	0.56	0.543
Own result	6.30		0.520

6.6 % by *Ph. Helvet.*, *Remington* and *Rosenthaler*, and 6.35 % by *Brit. Pharm. Codex*. We find it is 6.3 %.

Natrii benzoas.

Vapour pressure determinations were made af the following solutions of sodium benzoate. In table 78 the results are given in the corresponding freezing point depressions.

Table 78.

The concentration of sodium benzoate grammes/1000 millilitres	5.00	10.00	20.00	35.00
The corresponding freezing point depression in °C.	0.123	0.232	0.462	0.812

In table 79 a comparison is made between the values for sodium benzoate found by other authors, and our own values.

Table 79.

Author	The concentration in %	The freezing point depression	The freezing point depression found by us according to fig. 23
Brit. Pharm. Codex 1934, Ph. Helvet. and Remington	1.0	0.31	0.232
Rosenthaler	1.80	0.56	0.417
Own result	2.25		0.520

It will be seen from table 79 that our values are 25 % lower than those stated by *Brit. Pharm. Codex, Remington,* and *Rosenthaler.* We should, however, consider our own values to be more probable, since, according to table 51, the calculated isoosmotic concentration amounts to 2.169 %, and we find experimentally that it is 2.25, which gives an activity coefficient of 0.96, whereas it, calculated on the basis of *Rosenthaler*'s value, exceeds 1; it amounts to 1.205, which must be considered rather improbable.

In fig. 23 the values of tables 72, 73, 74, 76, and 78 have been marked in the same manner as the values in fig. 6.

Fig.23

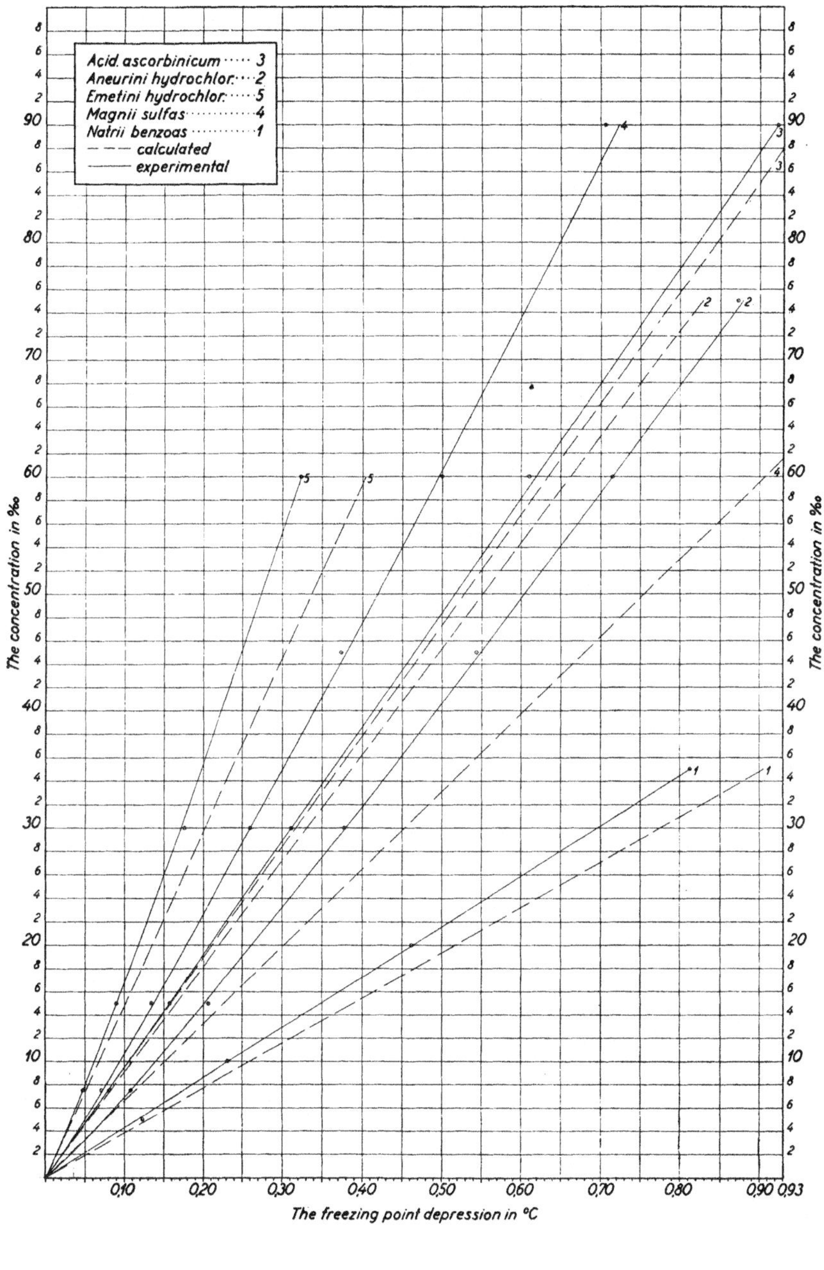
Acid. ascorbinicum ····· 3
Aneurini hydrochlor. ···· 2
Emetini hydrochlor. ····· 5
Magnii sulfas ············ 4
Natrii benzoas ··········· 1
calculated
experimental
The concentration in ‰
The freezing point depression in °C

Acidum citricum.

Vapour pressure determinations were made of the following solutions of citric acid. In table 80 the results are shown in the corresponding freezing point depressions.

Table 80.

The concentration of citric acid grammes/1000 millilitres	7.50	15.00	30.00	60.00	90.00
The corresponding freezing point depression in ^{0}C.	0.073	0.144	0.287	0.564	0.839

We have found no values in literature with which to compare our results.

Mersalylum.

Vapour pressure determinations were made of the following solutions of mersalyl. In table 81 the results are given in the corresponding freezing point depressions.

Table 81.

The concentration of mersalyl grammes/1000 millilitres	7.50	15.00	30.00	60.00	100.0
The corresponding freezing point depression in ^{0}C.	0.045	0.090	0.182	0.350	0.564

We have found no values in literature with which to compare our results.

Narcotini hydrochloridum.

Vapour pressure determinations were made of the following solutions of narcotine hydrochloride. In table 82 the results are given in the corresponding freezing point depressions.

Table 82.

The concentration of narcotine hydrochloride grammes/1000 millilitres	12.50	25.00	50.00	100.0
The corresponding freezing point depression in ^{0}C.	0.062	0.123	0.244	0.401

Our values differ somewhat from *Schou's*, as we find, with reference to fig. 24, that a 1 % solution of narcotine hydrochloride gives a freezing point depression of 0.056^0, whereas *Schou* states it to be 0.062^0.

Natrii salicylas.

Vapour pressure determinations were made of the following solutions of sodium salicylate. In table 83 the results are given in the corresponding freezing point depressions.

Table 83.

The concentration of sodium salicylate grammes/1000 millilitres	5.00	10.00	20.00	40.00
The corresponding freezing point depression in °C.	0.102	0.209	0.412	0.818

The obtained results agree well with the value given in *Remington*'s »*Practice of Pharmacy*« of a 0.22° freezing point depression in the case of a 1 % solution of sodium salicylate. In reference to fig. 24 we arrive at 0.209°.

Oxychinolini sulfas.

Vapour pressure determinations were made of the following solutions of potassium hydroxy quinolin sulphate. In table 84 the results are given in the corresponding freezing point depressions.

Table 84.

The concentration of potassium hydroxy quinolin sulphate grammes/1000 millilitres	5.00	10.00	20.00	40.00	70.00
The corresponding freezing point depression in °C.	0.084	0.159	0.275	0.502	0.840

We have found no results in literature with which to compare our values.

Pentazolum.

Vapour pressure determinations were made of the following solutions of leptazole. In table 85 the results are given in the corresponding freezing point depressions.

Table 85.

The concentration of leptazole grammes / 1000 millilitres	7.50	15.00	30.00	45.00	60.00	90.00	100.0
The corresponding freezing point depression	0.097	0.186	0.340	0.490	0.621	0.870	0.940

We have found no values in literature with which to compare our results.

In fig. 24 the values of tables 80, 81, 82, 83, 84, and 85 have been marked in the same manner as the values in fig. 6.

Fig. 24

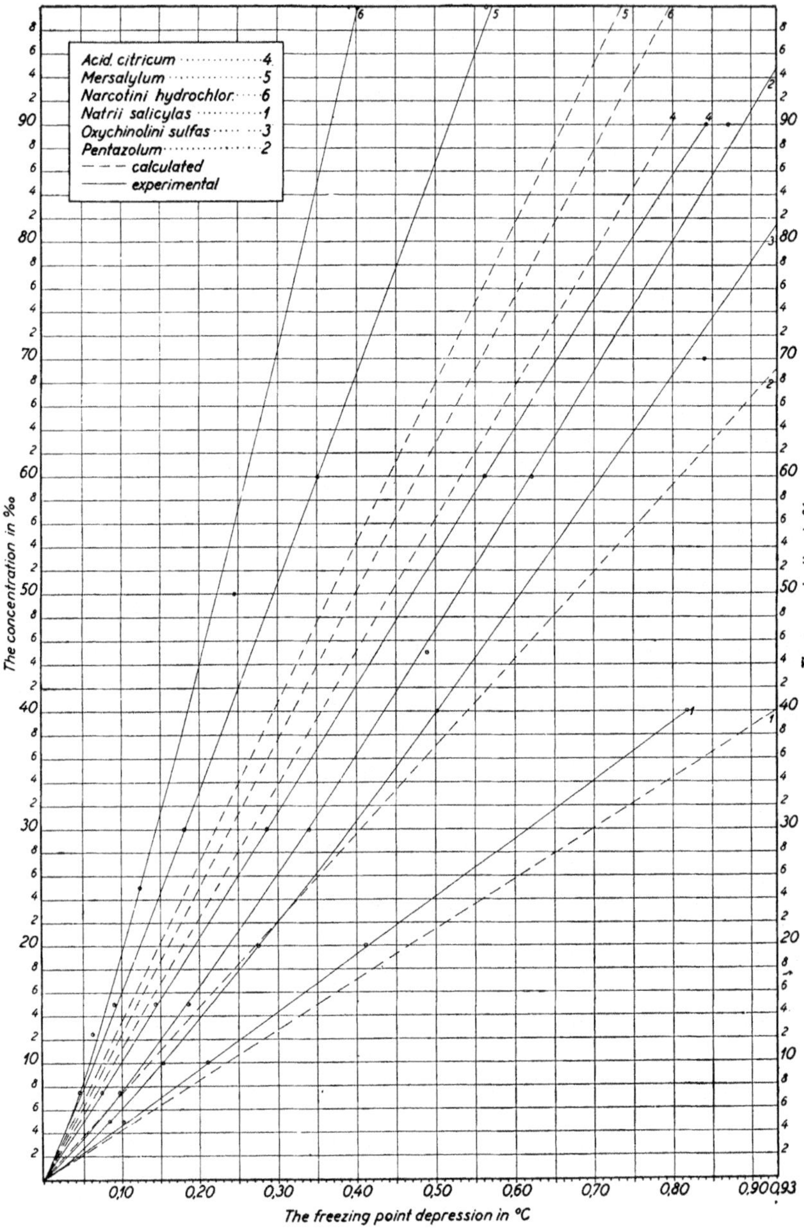
Acid. citricum 4
Mersalylum 5
Narcotini hydrochlor. 6
Natrii salicylas 1
Oxychinolini sulfas 3
Pentazolum 2
calculated
experimental
The concentration in ‰
The freezing point depression in °C

Chloraminum.

Freezing point determinations were made of the following solutions of chloramine. The results, which have been corrected as to the amount of disengaged ise (see p. 46), are given in table 86.

Table 86.

The concentration of chloramine grammes/1000 millilitres	10.00	20.00	50.00	60.00
The determined freezing point depression in °C.	0.133	0.255	0.635	0.750

As it is possible that solutions of chloramine may penetrate the insulating varnish coating of *Hill*'s thermo-element, and thus spoil the element, we have made these determinations through a direct measuring of the freezing point in *Beckmann*'s apparatus. It will be seen from fig. 25 that we find a 4.1 % solution of chloramine to be isoosmotic with blood.

Jodphtaleinum.

Freezing point determinations were made of the following solutions of soluble iodophthalein. The results, which have been corrected as to the amount of disengaged ice (see p. 46), are given in table 87.

Table 87.

The concentration of soluble iodophthalein grammes/ 1000 millilitres............	5.00	10.00	20.00	30.00	40.00	80.00	100.0
The determined freezing point depression in °C.	0.055	0.094	0.154	0.211	0.266	0.458	0.539

As it proved impossible to obtain reproducible values by means of the determination of the vapour pressure of the soluble iodophthalein solution, that method was abandoned. A direct determination of the freezing point depression, however, gave satisfactory results.

Mercuranum.

Vapour pressure determinations were made of the following solutions of merbromin. In table 88 the results are given in the corresponding freezing point depressions.

Table 88.

The concentration of merbromin grammes/1000 millilitres	12.50	25.00	50.00
The corresponding freezing point depression in ^{0}C.	0.097	0.159	0.274

We have found no results in literature with which to compare our values.

Natrii arsenas.

Vapour pressure determinations were made of the following solutions of sodium arsenate ($Na_2HAsO_4 \cdot 7H_2O$). In table 89 the results are given in the corresponding freezing point depressions.

Table 89.

The concentration of sodium arsenate grammes/1000 millilitres	5.00	10.00	20.00	40.00	60.00
The corresponding freezing point depression in ^{0}C.	0.076	0.141	0.278	0.540	0.798

Our values differ much from the one stated by *Schou,* who finds that a 1 % solution of sodium arsenate should correspond to a 0.3 % solution of sodium chloride, which gives a freezing point depression of 0.179^0, whereas we, in conformity with fig. 25, find it is 0.143^0.

Natrii jodidum.

Vapour pressure determinations were made of the following solutions of sodium iodide. In table 90 the results are given in the corresponding freezing point depressions.

Table 90.

The concentration of sodium iodide grammes/1000 millilitres	5.00	10.00	20.00	30.00	40.00
The corresponding freezing point depression in ^{0}C.	0.113	0.219	0.442	0.653	0.870

In table 91 a comparison has been made between the sodium iodide values of other authors and our own values.

Table 91.

Author	The concentration in %	The freezing point depression	The freezing point depression we find according to fig. 25
Landolt-Börnstein 1931	0.928	0.2027	0.207
» »	1.837	0.4325	0.406
Rosenthaler	2.50	0.56	0.584
Own result	2.37		0.520

It will be seen that there is a fairly good agreement between the values stated by ***Landolt-Börnstein*** and ***Rosenthaler,*** and our own values. The isoosmotic concentration is stated by ***Rosenthaler*** to be 2.50 %, we find 2.37 %.

Nicaethamidum.

Vapour pressure determinations were made of the following solutions of nikethamide. In table 92 the results are given in the corresponding freezing point depressions.

Table 92.

The concentration of nikethamide grammes/1000 millilitres	7.50	15.00	30.00	45.00	60.00	100.0
The corresponding freezing point depression in °C	0.072	0.148	0.279	0.404	0.518	0.816

We have found no values in literature with which to compare our results.

Tanninum.

Vapour pressure determinations were made of the following solutions of tannic acid. In table 93 the results are given in the corresponding freezing point depressions.

Table 93.

The concentration of tannic acid grammes/1000 millilitres	7.50	15.00	30.00	60.00	90.00	120.0
The corresponding freezing point depression in °C.	0.012	0.024	0.052	0.098	0.154	0.200

We have found no values in literature with which to compare our results.

In fig. 25 the values of tables 86, 87, 88, 89, 90, 92, and 93 have been marked in the same manner as the values in fig. 6.

Fig.25

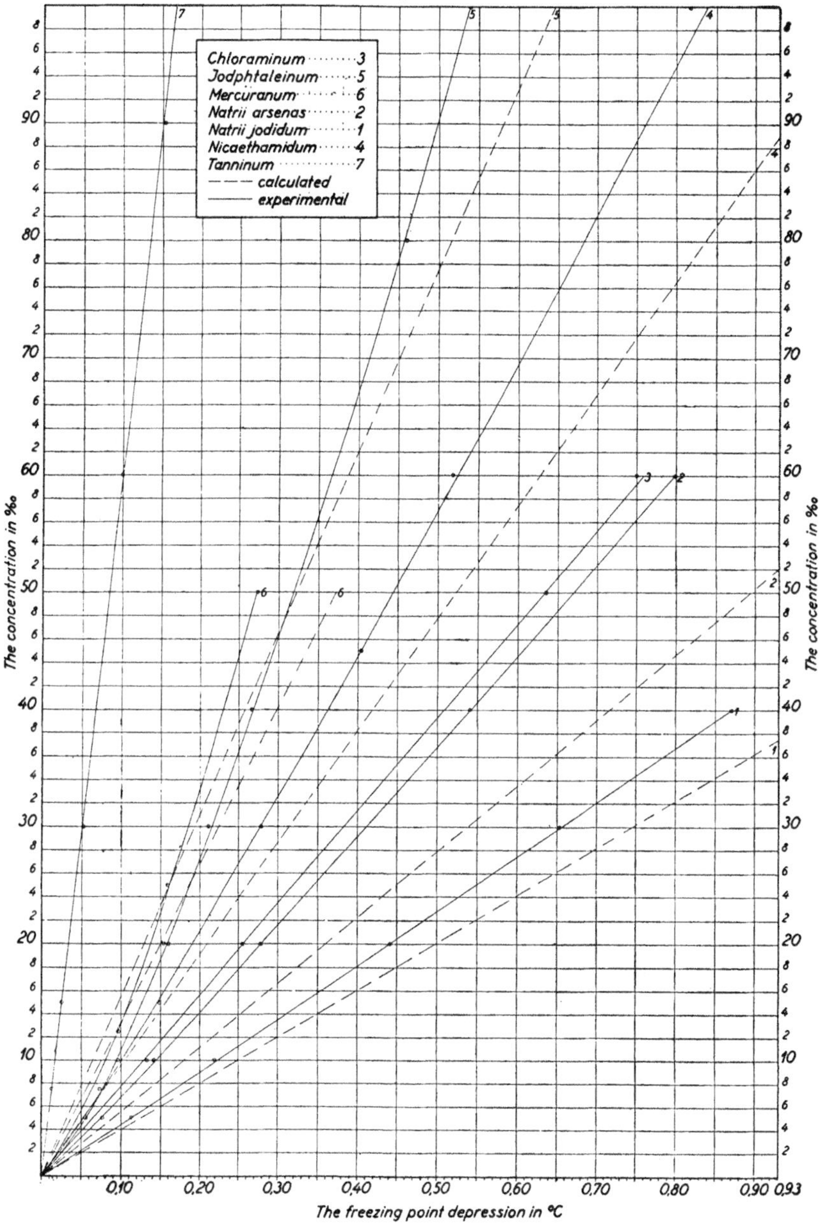

Chloraminum 3
Jodphtaleinum 5
Mercuranum 6
Natrii arsenas 2
Natrii jodidum 1
Nicaethamidum 4
Tanninum 7
calculated
experimental
The concentration in ‰
The freezing point depression in °C
0,10 0,20 0,30 0,40 0,50 0,60 0,70 0,80 0,90 0,93
10 20 30 40 50 60 70 80 90

Amphetamini sulfas.

Vapour pressure determinations were made of the following solutions of amphetamine sulphate. In table 94 the results are given in the corresponding freezing point depressions.

Table 94.

The concentration of amphetamine sulphate grammes/1000 millilitres	7.50	15.00	30.00	60.00
The corresponding freezing point depression in °C.	0.097	0.191	0.371	0.728

We have found no values in literature with which to compare our results.

Cincaini hydrochloridum.

Vapour pressure determinations were made of the following solutions of cinchocaine hydrochloride. In table 95 the results are given in the corresponding freezing point depressions.

Table 95.

The concentration of cinchocaine hydrochloride grammes/1000 millilitres	5.00	7.50	10.00	15.00	20.00	30.00	40.00	45.00	60.00	80.00	120.0
The corresponding freezing point depression in °C. ..	0.040	0.056	0.076	0.106	0.139	0.188	0.210	0.222	0.235	0.253	0.294

Our values differ somewhat from *Schou*'s, according to whom a 1 % solution of cinchocaine hydrochloride should correspond to a 0.13 % solution of sodium chloride, which gives a freezing point depression of 0.079°, whereas we, according to fig. 26, find 0.074°.

Natrii phosphas.

Vapour pressure determinations were made of the following solutions of disodium hydrogen phosphate — 2 H_2O. In table 96 the concentrations employed have been converted into the corresponding concentrations of disodium hydrogen phosphate with water of crystallisation of 7 and 12 molecules respectively. The results of the vapour pressure determinations are shown in table 96 in the corresponding freezing point depressions.

Table 96

The concentration of Na_2HPO_4, $2H_2O$ grammes/1000 millilitres	7.50	15.00	20.00	30.00	35.00
Na_2HPO_4, $7H_2O$ grammes/1000 millilitres	11.28	22.56	30.10	45.13	52.65
Na_2HPO_4, $12H_2O$ grammes/1000 millilitres	15.09	30.18	40.23	60.35	70.41
The corresponding freezing point depression in ^0C.	0.184	0.395	0.473	0.692	0.793

In table 97 a comparison has been made between other authors' values of sodium phosphate (Na_2HPO_4, $12\ H_2O$), and our own values.

Table 97.

Author	The concentration in %	The freezing point depression	The freezing point depression we find according to fig. 26
Böhme	0.38	0.05	0.050
»	0.78	0.10	0.100
»	1.13	0.15	0.142
»	1.51	0.20	0.187
»	1.92	0.25	0.235
»	2.34	0.30	0.285
»	2.75	0.35	0.330
»	3.18	0.40	0.379
»	3.60	0.45	0.426
»	4.01	0.50	0.471
Brit. Pharm. Codex and Remington	4.53	0.56	0.529
Rosenthaler	4.50	0.56	0.525
»	6.45	0.80	0.737
Own result	4.45		0.520

It will be seen from table 97 that there is a good agreement between other authors' values of sodium phosphate, and our own values. Thus the isoosmotic concentration is stated by ***Brit. Pharm. Codex,*** and ***Remington*** to be 4.53 %, by ***Rosenthaler*** 4.50 %, and we find 4.45 %.

Natrii thiosulfas.

Vapour pressure determinations were made of the following solutions of sodium thiosulphate. In table 98 the results are given in the corresponding freezing point depressions.

Table 98.

The concentration of sodium thiosulphate grammes/1000 millilitres	5.00	10.00	20.00	30.00	40.00	50.00
The corresponding freezing point depression in °C.	0.092	0.180	0.354	0.524	0.692	0.846

There is a good agreement between our results and the result stated in *Remington*'s »*Practice of Pharmacy*« of a freezing point depression of 0.178° in the case of a solution of 1 %; the same is true about *Landolt-Börnstein,* stating that a solution of 5.021 % has a freezing point depression of 0.855°, while we, according to fig. 26, arrive at 0.180° and 0.862° in the case of solutions of 1 % and 5.021 % respectively.

Procaini hydrochloridum.

Vapour pressure determinations were made of the following solutions of procaine hydrochloride. In table 99 the results are given in the corresponding freezing point depressions.

Table 99.

The concentration of procaine hydrochloride grammes/1000 millilitres	7.50	15.00	30.00	45.00	60.00	90.00
The corresponding freezing point depression in °C.	0.091	0.179	0.333	0.468	0.610	0.848

In table 100 a comparison has been made between other authors' procaine hydrochloride values and our own values.

It will be seen in table 100 that there is a great disagreement between the values of the various authors. Thus *Schou*'s value is about 10 % lower than ours, whereas *Brit. Pharm. Codex, Ph. Helvet., Remington, Böhme,* and *Rosenthaler* all of them generally find much higher (up to 20—25 %) freezing point depressions than we find. The isoosmotic concentration is stated by *Rosenthaler* to be 4.45 %, by *Remington* to be 5.0 %; we find it is 5.05 %.

Ph. Norv. states that 0.72, 0.54, and 0.36 % of sodium chloride must be added to 3 solutions of procaine hydrochloride of 1, 2, and 3 % respectively, in order to obtain isoosmosis; we find that the percentage of sodium chloride should be 0.69, 0.50, and 0.32 respectively.

Table 100.

Author	The concentration in %	The freezing point depression	The freezing point depression we find according to fig. 26
Schou	1.0	0.109	0.122
Brit. Pharm. Codex 1934, Ph. Helvet., Remington, and van Itallie	1.0	0.14	0.122
Ph. Helvet., Remington, and van Itallie	2.0	0.25	0.227
Remington	5.0	0.56	0.515
Own result	5.05		0.520
Rosenthaler	4.45	0.56	0.464
»	6.40	0.80	0.643
Böhme	0.559	0.092	0.071
»	1.071	0.160	0.129
»	1.604	0.222	0.186
»	2.046	0.264	0.231
»	2.763	0.352	0.304

Tetracaini hydrochloridum.

Vapour pressure determinations were made of the following solutions of amethocaine hydrochloride. In table 101 the results are given in the corresponding freezing point depressions.

Table 101.

The concentration of amethocaine hydrochloride grammes/1000 millilitres	5.00	7.50	10.00	15.00	20.00	30.00	40.00	45.00	60.00	80.00	100.0
The corresponding freezing point depression in °C.	0.061	0.086	0.110	0.150	0.191	0.261	0.324	0.341	0.383	0.445	0.485

Our values differ considerably from *Schou's*, who states that a 1 % solution of amethocaine hydrochloride should correspond to a 0.13 % solution of sodium chloride, which gives a freezing point depression of 0.074°, whereas we, according to fig. 26, arrive at 0.109°.

In fig. 26 the values from tables 94, 95, 96, 98, 99, and 101 have been marked in a similar manner as the values in fig. 6.

Fig.26

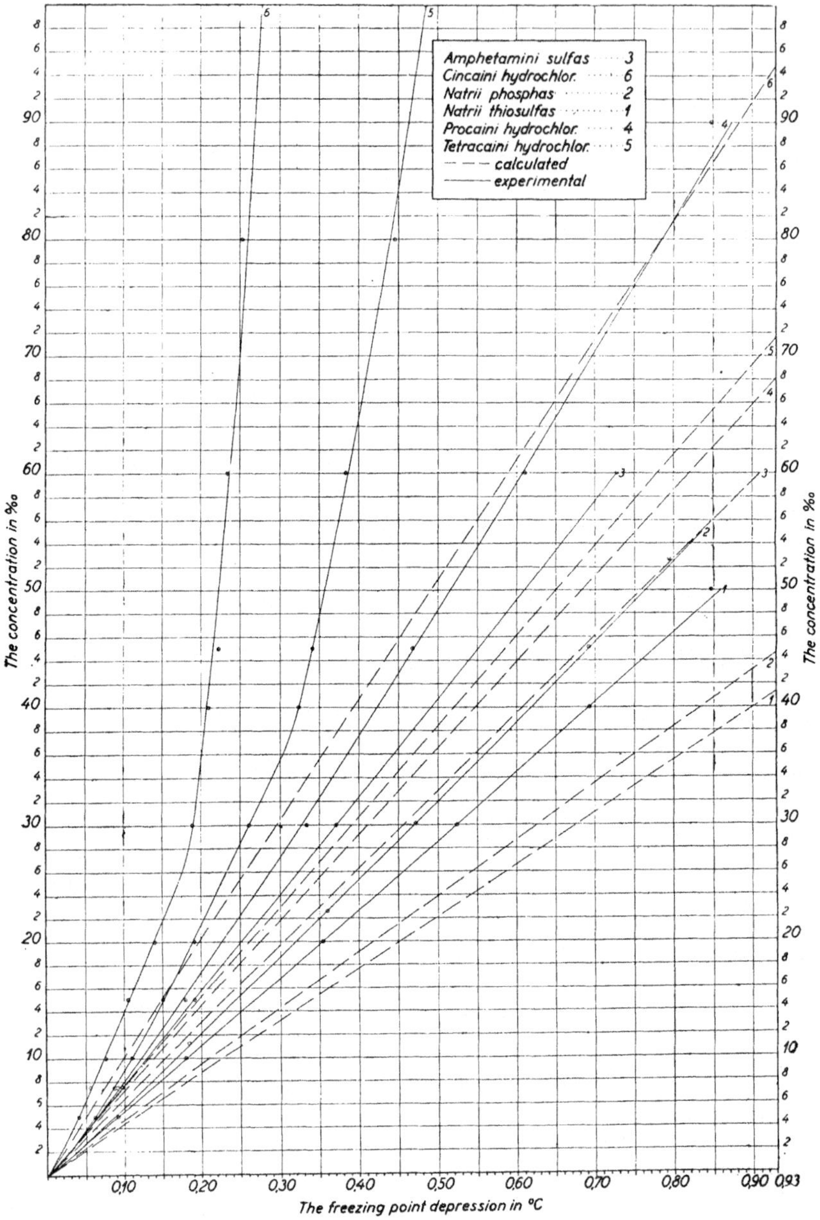
Amphetamini sulfas 3
Cincaini hydrochlor. 6
Natrii phosphas 2
Natrii thiosulfas 1
Procaini hydrochlor. 4
Tetracaini hydrochlor. 5
calculated
experimental
The concentration in ‰
The freezing point depression in °C

Acidum nicotinicum.

Vapour pressure determinations were made of the following solutions of nicotinic acid. In table 102 the results are given in the corresponding freezing point depressions.

Table 102.

The concentration of nicotinic acid grammes/1000 millilitres	5.00	10.00	12.50
The corresponding freezing point depression in °C.	0.074	0.145	0.180

We have found no values in literature with which to compare our result.

Calcii gluconas.

Vapour pressure determinations were made of the following solutions of calcium gluconate. In table 103 the results are given the corresponding freezing point depressions.

Table 103.

The concentration of calcium gluconate grammes/1000 millilitres	7.50	15.00	30.00
The corresponding freezing point depression in °C.	0.071	0.131	0.237

Our values differ considerably from the freezing point depression of 0.054° in the case of a 1 % solution, as stated in *Remington*'s »*Practice of Pharmacy*«. According to fig. 27 we find 0.091°.

Chinini hydrochloridum.

Vapour pressure determinations were made of the following solutions of quinine hydrochloride. In table 104 the results are given in the corresponding freezing point depressions.

Table 104.

The concentration of quinine hydrochloride grammes/1000 millilitres	7.50	15.00	30.00
The corresponding freezing point depression in °C.	0.059	0.111	0.194

The results given in table 104 agree well with the value stated by *Schou*, that a 1 % solution of quinine hydrochloride corresponds to a 0.13 % solution of sodium chloride, which gives a freezing point depression of 0.079°, while we, according to fig. 27, arrive at 0.077°.

There is also a good agreement with *Ph. Norv.* stating that 0.77 % of sodium chloride must be added to a 1 % solution of quinine hydrochloride to obtain isoosmosis; we find 0.76 %.

Ephedrini hydrochloridum.

Vapour pressure determinations were made of the following solutions of ephedrine hydrochloride. In table 105 the results are given in the corresponding freezing point depressions.

Table 105.

The concentration of ephedrine hydrochloride grammes/1000 millilitres	6.25	12.50	25.00	50.00
The corresponding freezing point depression in °C.	0.111	0.208	0.403	0.807

In table 106 a comparison is made between the ephedrine hydrochloride values of others, and our own values.

Table 106.

Author	The concentration in %	The freezing point depression	The freezing point depression we find according to fig. 27
Schou	1	0.162	0.169
Rosenthaler	4.05	0.56	0.653
»	5.80	0.80	0.920
Own result	3.20		0.520

It will be seen from the values in table 106 that there is a good agreement between *Schou*'s value and our own ones. *Rosenthaler*'s freezing point depression, on the other hand, lies about 13 or 14 % lower than our values. The isoosmotic concentration is stated to be 4.5 % by *Rosenthaler*, whereas we find 3.20 %.

Ferrosi lactas.

Vapour pressure determinations were made of the following solutions of ferrous lactate. In table 107 the results are given in the corresponding freezing point depressions.

Table 107.

The concentration of ferrous lactate grammes/1000 millilitres	5.00	10.00	20.00
The corresponding freezing point depression in °C.	0.062	0.121	0.237

We have found no values in literature with which to compare our results.

Glycerinum.

Vapour pressure determinations were made of the following solutions of glycerin. In table 108 the results are given in the corresponding freezing point depressions.

Table 108.

The concentration of glycerin grammes/1000 millilitres	5.00	10.00	20.00	40 00
The corresponding freezing point depression in °C.	0.104	0.204	0.403	0.799

In table 109 a comparison has been made between the glycerin values of other authors, and our own values.

Table 109.

Author	The concentration in %	The freezing point depression	The freezing point depression we find according to fig. 27
Landolt-Börnstein 1923	0.1841	0.0372	0.038
» »	0.9280	0.1869	0.190
» »	2.042	0.4140	0.403
Landolt-Börnstein 1927	1.164	0.2338	0.237
» »	2.594	0.5285	0.520
Rosenthaler	3.95	0.80	0.786
Own result	2.60		0.520

It will be seen that there is a good agreement between the values stated by others, and those found by us.

As to the freezing point depression of mixtures of glycerin and water, see fig. 40 of this treatise.

Lobelini hydrochloridum.

Vapour pressure determinations were made of the following solutions of lobeline hydrochloride. In table 110 the results are given in the corresponding freezing point depressions.

Table 110.

The concentration of lobeline hydrochloride grammes/1000 millilitres	5.00	10.00	20.00
The corresponding freezing point depression in °C.	0.047	0.091	0.174

The values given in table 110 differ much from the value stated by *Schou*, that a 1 % solution of lobeline hydrochloride should correspond to a 0.13 % solution of sodium chloride, which gives a freezing point depression of 0.079°, whereas we, according to fig. 27, find it is 0.092°.

Natrii bicarbonas.

Vapour pressure determinations were made of the following solutions of sodium bicarbonate. In table 111 the results are given in the corresponding freezing point depressions.

Table 111.

The concentration of sodium bicarbonate grammes/1000 millilitres	5.00	10.00	15.00	20.00
The corresponding freezing point depression in °C.	0.197	0.375	0.561	0.732

In table 112 a comparison is made between the sodium bicarbonate values of other authors, and our own values.

Table 112.

Author	The concentration in %	The freezing point depression	The freezing point depression we find according to fig. 27
Brit. Pharm. Codex 1934	1.0	0.40	0.381
» »	1.35	0.56	0.505
» »	2.00	0.86	0.738
Landolt-Börnstein 1923	0.985	0.420	0.377
Remington and Ph. Helvet...	1.0	0.40	0.381
» » ..	1.4	0.56	0.523

Table 112 (continued).

Author	The concentration in %	The freezing point depression	The freezing point depression we find according to fig. 27
Remington and Ph. Helvet...	2.0	0.80	0.738
Böhme	0.59	0.25	0.230
»	0.83	0.35	0.320
»	1.08	0.45	0.410
»	1.33	0.55	0.498
»	1.57	0.65	0.584
»	1.84	0.75	0.680
Rosenthaler	1.35	0.56	0.505
»	1,95	0.80	0.719
Own result	1.39		0.520

Even if our values, according to table 112, on the whole show slightly lower freezing point depressions than do the values of the other authors, there is a good agreement in the statements of the isoosmotic concentration, which is stated by *Ph. Helvet.* and *Remington* to be 1.4 %, by *Brit. Pharm. Codex* and by *Rosenthaler* 1.35 %, and we find 1.39 %. It may be added that we have repeatedly found a freezing point depression of 0.52° (which is the corrected result) in the case of a 1.4 % solution of sodium bicarbonate. Thus it will be seen that solutio natrii bicarbonatis isotonica (Dispensatorium Danicum), which contains 1.3 % of sodium bicarbonate, corresponding to the calculated isoosmotic concentration, is slightly hypotonic.

Natrii citras.

The following measurements of sodium citrate ($C_6H_5O_7Na_3$ $2H_2O$) were made partly by freezing point determinations, partly by vapour pressure determinations. The results are shown in table 113; in the case of the vapour pressure determinations they are given in the corresponding freezing point depressions.

Table 113.

The concentration of sodium citrate grammes/1000 millilitres	5.00	10.00	20.00	30.00	40.00	50.00
The freezing point depression in °C.	0.090	0.181	0.366	0.516	0.697	0.825
Vapour pressure determination ..	0.089	0.178	0.351	0.519	0.682	0.825

It will be seen from table 113 that good agreement has been found between the values arrived at in a direct manner by means of a determination of the freezing point depression, and the values found indirectly by means of a determination of the vapour pressure. As sodium citrate is the only substance examined in this part of the treatise of which we have made determinations by means of both the methods employed, the results obtained, which agree well, emphasize the justification for the comparison made. It must be emphasized that agreement has been reached, even though the freezing point determinations have been made at a temperature of about 0°, and the vapour pressure determinations at 20°.

In table 114 a comparison is made between the sodium citrate values of other authors, and our own values.

Table 114.

Author	The concentration in %	The freezing point depression	The freezing point depression we find according to fig. 27
Warburg	0.723	0.146	0.130
»	1.450	0.274	0.255
»	2.166	0.401	0.377
»	2.890	0.519	0.499
Schou	2.3	0.56	0.399
Remington	1.0	0.224	0.178
»	2.5	0.449	0.433
Own result	3.02		0.520

It will be seen from table 114 that *Warburg*'s freezing point depressions are between 4 and 7 % higher than our own ones; yet there is a still greater difference in the case of the lowest concentrations, where *Warburg*'s value is 12 % higher than ours.

Comparing the values of tables 114 and 51 it will be seen that *Schou's* statement of the isoosmotic concentration is very near to the calculated value, but on the other hand *Schou*'s value, expressed in freezing point depression, is about 40 % higher than our experimentally found value. One of *Remington*'s values agrees well with ours, the other value is about 25 % higher than ours, which fact indicates that the first *Remington* value has been found experimentally, and that the second value is merely a calculated one.

It is very unfortunate when the same table contains two values which are mutually so disagreeing that it may be difficult to decide which of them to use. This is seen clearly, if the isoosmotic concentration is calculated on the basis of the values in table 114.

Schou	2.3 %
Remington	2.5 %
»	3.1 %
Warburg	2.6 %
»	2.8 %
»	2.8 %
»	2.9 %
Own result ...	3.0 %

Papaverini hydrochloridum.

Vapour pressure determinations were made of the following solutions of papaverine hydrochloride. In table 115 the results are given in the corresponding freezing point depressions.

Table 115.

The concentration of papaverine hydrochloride grammes/1000 millilitres	5.00	10.00	20.00
The corresponding freezing point depression in °C.	0.028	0.062	0.121

Our values differ considerably from the one stated by *Schou,* according to whom a 1 % solution of papaverine hydrochloride should correspond to a 0.13 % solution of sodium chloride, which gives a freezing point depression of 0.079°, whereas we, according to fig. 27, find it is 0.062°.

In fig. 27 the values from tables 102, 103, 104, 105, 107, 108, 110, 111, 113, and 115 have been marked in the same manner as the values in fig. 6.

Fig.27

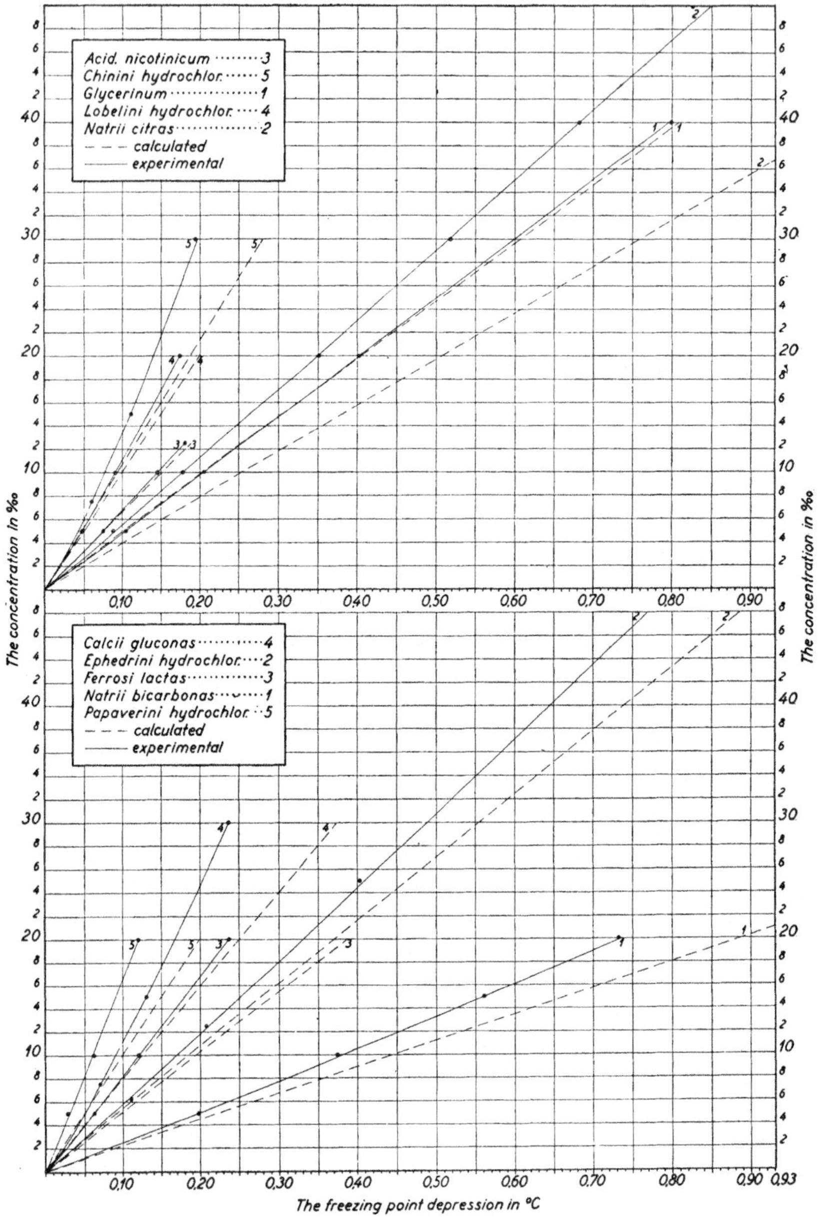
Acid. nicotinicum ········3
Chinini hydrochlor. ······5
Glycerinum ···············1
Lobelini hydrochlor. ····4
Natrii citras ·············2
– – – calculated
——— experimental
Calcii gluconas ···········4
Ephedrini hydrochlor. ···2
Ferrosi lactas ·············3
Natrii bicarbonas ········1
Papaverini hydrochlor. ··5
– – – calculated
——— experimental
The concentration in ‰
The freezing point depression in °C
0,10
0,20
0,30
0,40
0,50
0,60
0,70
0,80
0,90
0,93
10
20
30
40

Apomorphini hydrochloridum.

Vapour pressure determinations were made of the following solutions of apomorphine hydrochloride. In table 116 the results are given in the corresponding freezing point depressions.

Table 116.

The concentration of apomorphine hydrochloride grammes/1000 millilitres	5.00	10.00	20.00
The corresponding freezing point depression in ^{0}C.	0.041	0.080	0.155

Our results differ much from the value stated by *Schou*, according to whom a 1 % solution of apomorphine hydrochloride should correspond to a 0.15 % solution of sodium chloride, which gives a freezing point depression of 0.091^0, whereas we, according to fig. 28, find it is 0.080^0. On the other hand there is a good agreement with *Ph. Norv.*, stating that 0.75 % of sodium chloride must be added to a 1 % solution of apomorphine hydrochloride to obtain isoosmosis; we find 0.755 %.

Calcii chloridum.

Vapour pressure determinations were made of the following solutions of calcium chloride. In table 117 the results are given in the corresponding freezing point depressions.

Table 117.

The concentration of calcium chloride grammes/1000 millilitres	5.00	10.00	20.00	30.00	40.00
The corresponding freezing point depression in ^{0}C.	0.093	0.200	0.421	0.636	0.853

In table 118 a comparison has been made between the values of calcium chloride found by other authors, and our own values.

Table 118.

Author	The concentration in %	The freezing point depression	The freezing point depression we find according to fig. 28
Landolt-Börnstein	1.1009	0.2437	0.221
» »	2.204	0.4823	0.458
Brit. Pharm. Codex and Remington	2.33	0.56	0.485
Own result	2.50		0.520

There is some disagreement between the calcium chloride values stated by others, and the values we have found. *Brit. Pharm. Codex* and *Remington* state the isoosmotic value to be 2.33 % ; we find it is 2.50 %.

Codeini hydrochloridum.

Vapour pressure determinations were made of the following solutions of codeine hydrochloride. In table 119 the results are given in the corresponding freezing point depressions.

Table 119.

The concentration of codeine hydrochloride grammes/1000 millilitres	7.50	15.00	30.00
The corresponding freezing point depression in °C.	0.066	0.129	0.253

The values given in table 119 agree well with the value stated by *Schou,* that a 1 % solution of codeine hydrochloride corresponds to a 0.14 % solution of sodium chloride, which gives a freezing point depression of 0.086°, while we, according to fig. 28, find it is 0.087°.

Diemalnatrium.

Vapour pressure determinations were made of the following solutions of soluble barbitone. In table 120 the results are given in the corresponding freezing point depressions.

Table 120.

The concentration of soluble barbitone grammes/1000 millilitres	5.00	10.00	20.00	40.00	50.00
The corresponding freezing point depression in °C.	0.082	0.172	0.337	0.661	0.822

We have found no values in literature with which to compare our results.

Kalii chloridum.

Vapour pressure determinations were made of the following solutions of potassium chloride. In table 121 the results are given in the corresponding freezing point depressions.

Table 121.

The concentration of potassium chloride grammes/1000 millilitres	5.00	10.00	15.00	20.00
The corresponding freezing point depression in ^{0}C.	0.219	0.439	0.656	0.868

In table 122 a comparison is made between the potassium chloride values of others, and our own results.

Table 122.

Author	The concentration in %	The freezing point depression	The freezing point depression found by us according to fig. 28
Landolt-Börnstein 1923	0.7042	0.3280	0.309
» »	1.559	0.705	0.682
Landolt-Börnstein 1927	0.7367	0.340	0.320
» »	0.9290	0.425	0.408
» »	1.5837	0.7164	0.692
» »	2.02	0.913	-0.883
Böhme	0.43	0.20	0.189
»	0.65	0.30	0.285
»	0.87	0.40	0.382
»	1.09	0.50	0.478
»	1.32	0.60	0.578
»	1.54	0.70	0.673
»	1.77	0.80	0.774
Remington	1.12	0.56	0.492
Rosenthaler	1.20	0.56	0.526
»	1.75	0.80	0.765
Warburg	0.559	0.236	0.244
»	1.118	0.516	0.490
»	1.680	0.763	0.735
Own result	1.19		0.520

It will be seen that there is a fairly good agreement between the values of the various authors and our own values. The concentration of the isoosmotic solution is stated by ***Remington*** to be 1.12 %, by ***Rosenthaler*** 1.20 %, and we find it is 1.19 %.

Kalii phosphas. (Sørensen's primary phosphate).

Vapour pressure determinations were made of the following solutions of potassium dihydrogen phosphate (KH_2PO_4). In table 123 the results are given in the corresponding freezing point depressions.

Table 123.

The concentration of potassium dihydrogen phosphate grammes/1000 millilitres	7.50	15.00	20.00	30.00	35.00
The corresponding freezing point depression in ^{0}C.	0.188	0.367	0.480	0.697	0.798

In table 124 a comparison is made between the values of potassium dihydrogen phosphate found by other authors, and those found by us.

Table 124.

Author	The concentration in %	The freezing point depression	The freezing point depression we find according to fig. 28
Landolt-Börnstein	0.2730	0.0720	0.076
» »	0.6834	0.1740	0.178
» »	2.751	0.6434	0.643
» »	0.751	0.186	0.193
» »	1.525	0.381	0.372
» »	3.506	0.809	0.806
Warburg	1.021	0.262	0.258
»	2.042	0.494	0.489
»	3.063	0.719	0.710
Own result	2.18		0.520

In table 124 very good agreement is seen between *Landolt-Börnstein*'s, *Warburg*'s, and our own values.

Natrii phosphas (Sørensen's secondary phosphate).

Vapour pressure determinations were made of the following solutions of disodium hydrogen phosphate with 2 molecules of water of crystallisation ($Na_2HPO_4 \cdot 2H_2O$). In table 125 the results are given in the corresponding freezing point depressions.

Table 125.

The concentration of $Na_2HPO_4 \cdot 2H_2O$ grammes/1000 millilitres	7.50	15.00	20.00	30.00	35.00
The corresponding freezing point depression in ^{0}C.	0.184	0.359	0.473	0.692	0.793

In table 126 a comparison is made between the values of disodium hydrogen phosphate found by other authors, and the values found by us.

Table 126.

Author	The concentration in %	The freezing point depression	The freezing point depression we find according to fig. 28
Landolt-Börnstein 1923	0.3568	0.0969	0.092
» »	0.8921	0.2304	0.219
» »	1.785	0.4345	0.422
Landolt-Börnstein 1931	0.381	0.100	0.098
» »	0.919	0.240	0.225
» »	1.745	0.435	0.413
» »	1.995	0.495	0.470
Warburg	1.184	0.302	0.286
»	1.780	0.437	0.421
Own result	2.23		0.520

It will be seen that there is good agreement in table 126 between *Landolt-Börnstein*'s, *Warburg*'s, and our own values.

Theophyllinum.

Vapour pressure determinations were made of the following solution of theophylline. In table 127 the result is given in the corresponding freezing point depression.

Table 127.

The concentration of theophylline grammes/1000 millilitres	5.00
The corresponding freezing point depression in °C.	0.028

It has not been possible to carry out determination of theophylline concentrations stronger than 0.5 %, because of its slight solubility in water.

We have found no values with which to compare our result.

Urethanum.

Vapour pressure determinations were made of the following solutions of urethane. In table 128 the results are given in the corresponding freezing point depressions.

Table 128.

The concentration of urethane grammes/1000 millilitres	5.00	10.00	20.00	30.00	40.00
The corresponding freezing point depression in ^{0}C.	0.088	0.178	0.355	0.538	0.697

There is a considerable disagreement between *Landolt-Börnstein*'s freezing point depression of 0.436^0 in the case of a solution of 2.085 %, and our own value of 0.370^0.

In fig. 28 the values of tables 116, 117, 119, 120, 121, 123, 125, 127, and 128 have been marked in the same manner as the values in fig. 6.

Fig. 28

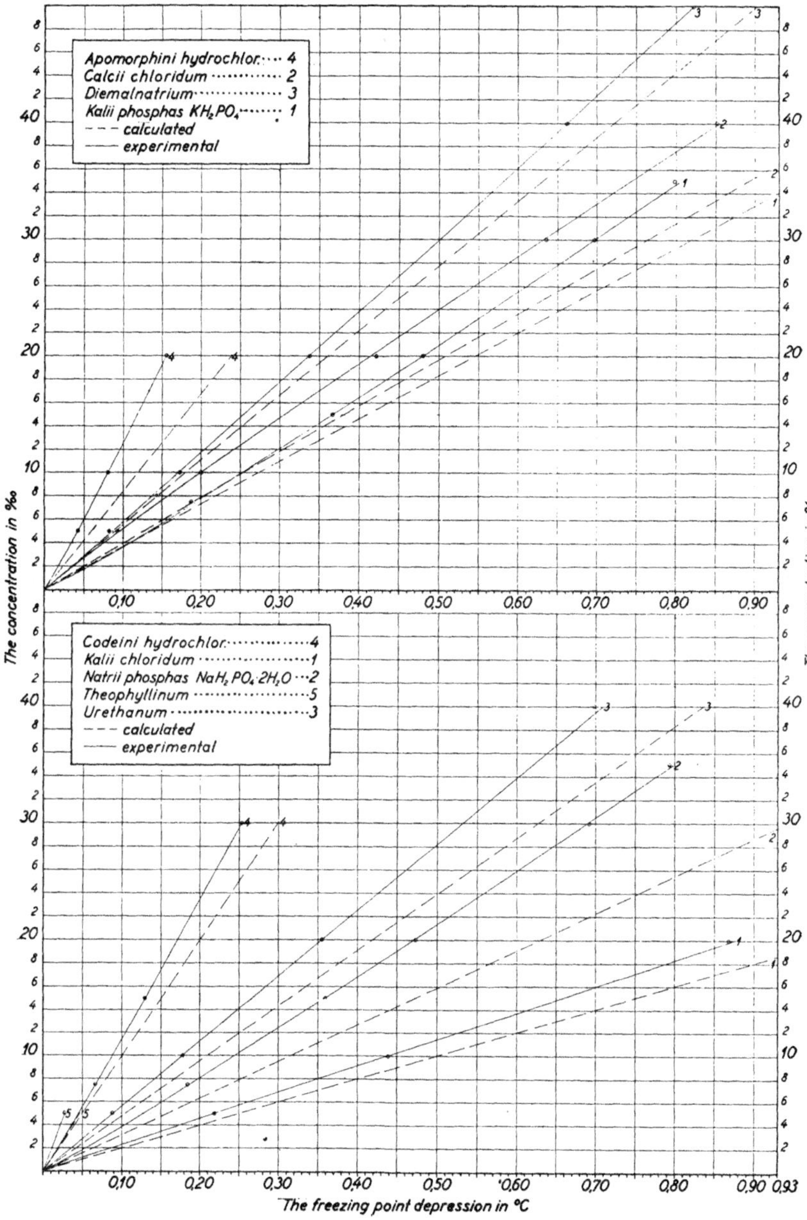
Apomorphini hydrochlor. 4
Calcii chloridum 2
Diemalnatrium 3
Kalii phosphas KH_2PO_4 1
calculated
experimental
Codeini hydrochlor. 4
Kalii chloridum 1
Natrii phosphas $NaH_2PO_4 \cdot 2H_2O$ 2
Theophyllinum 5
Urethanum 3
calculated
experimental
The concentration in ‰
The freezing point depression in °C

Aethylendiamini hydras.

Vapour pressure determinations were made of the following solutions of ethylene diamine. In table 129 the results are given in the corresponding freezing point depressions.

Table 129.

The concentration of ethylene diamine grammes/1000 millilitres	5.00	10.00	20.00
The corresponding freezing point depression in °C.	0.130	0.248	0.501

We have found no values in literature with which to compare our results.

Arseni trioxydum.

Vapour pressure determinations were made of the following solutions of arsenic trioxide. In table 130 the results are given in the corresponding freezing point depressions.

Table 130.

The concentration of arsenic trioxide grammes/1000 millilitres	4.81	9.92
The corresponding freezing point depression in °C.	0.082	0.168

In table 131 a comparison is made between the values of arsenic trioxide found by other authors, and the values found by us.

Table 131.

Author	The concentration in %	The freezing point depression	The freezing point depression found by us according to fig. 29
Landolt-Börnstein	0.1828	0.0335	0.031
» »	0.3684	0.0680	0.062
» »	0.4738	0.0870	0.081

According to table 131 *Landolt-Börnstein* states a freezing point depression which is 8 to 10 % greater than the one which we find.

Euflavinum.

Freezing point determinations were made of the following solutions of euflavine. The results, which have been corrected as to the amount af disengaged ice, p. 46, are shown in table 132.

Table 132.

The concentration of euflavine grammes/1000 millilitres	5.00	10.00	20.00	30.00
The determined freezing point depression in °C.	0.025	0.045	0.099	0.151

As euflavine seemed to affect the insulating varnish covering of *Hill*'s thermo-element, we have in this case made direct determinations of the freezing point depression in *Beckmann*'s apparatus.

We have found no values in literature with which to compare our results.

Hexamethylentetraminum.

Vapour pressure determinations were made of the following solutions of hexamine (methenamine). In table 133 the results are given in the corresponding freezing point depressions.

Table 133.

The concentration of hexamine grammes/1000 millilitres	7.50	15.00	30.00	50.00	60.00
The corresponding freezing point depression in °C.	0.100	0.199	0.415	0.724	0.879

Our results differ much from the value given by *Schou,* according to whom a 1 % solution of hexamine should correspond to a 0.19 % solution of sodium chloride, which gives a freezing point depression of 0.115°, whereas we, according to fig. 29, arrive at 0.129°.

Kalii permanganas.

Vapour pressure determinations were made of the following solutions of potassium permanganate. In table 134 the results are given in the corresponding freezing point depressions.

Table 134.

The concentration of potassium permanganate grammes/1000 millilitres	5.00	10.00	20.00
The corresponding freezing point depression in °C.	0.112	0.228	0.449

We have found no values in literature with which to compare our results.

The isoosmotic concentration is, according to our determinations, 2.3 %. (Fig. 29).

Morphini hydrochloridum.

Vapour pressure determinations were made of the following solutions of morphine hydrochloride. In table 135 the results are given in the corresponding freezing point depressions.

Table 135.

The concentration of morphini hydrochloride grammes/1000 millilitres	7.50	15.00	30.00
The corresponding freezing point depression in °C.	0.064	0.127	0.248

In table 136 we have compared the morphine hydrochloride values of other authors with our own values.

Table 136.

Author	The concentration in %	The freezing point depression	The freezing point depression we find according to fig. 29
Schou	1.0	0.079	0.086
Brit. Pharm. Codex 1934 ..	1.0	0.096	0.086
Ph. Helvet., Remington, and van Italie	1.0	0.096	0.086
»	2.0	0.185	0.168
»	3.0	0.273	0.248
Rosenthaler	6.95	0.56	
»	9.90	0.80	

It will be seen from table 136 that our morphine hydrochloride values are much higher than *Schou's*, and much lower than *van Itallie's*, *Ph. Helvet.'s*, and *Remington's.* As to the concentrations stated by *Rosenthaler,* it seems strange that it should have been possible to determine the freezing point of solutions of so strong concentrations. The solubility of morphine hydrochloride in water is stated in *Ph. Gall.* to be 50 % at 100°, and 4 % at 15°. Nevertheless *Rosenthaler's* isoosmotic concentration of 6.95 % corresponds well with the one of 7 % that we arrive at by extending the straight line that in the logarithmic system goes through our three observations, to the freezing point depression of 0.52°. *Ph. Norv.* states that 0.77, 0.64, and 0.51 % of sodium chloride must be added to 3 solutions of morphine hydrochloride of 1, 2, and 3 % respectively, to obtain isoosmosis; we find the slightly lower sodium chloride values of 0.74, 0.60, and 0.47 % respectively.

Phenolum.

Determinations of the vapour pressure and the freezing point depression were made of the following solutions of phenol. The results are given in table 137. The results of the freezing point determinations have been corrected as to the amount of disengaged ice.

Table 137.

The concentration of phenol grammes/1000 millilitres ..	5.00	10.00	20.00	30.00	40.00	50.00
Vapour pressure determination, given in the corresponding freezing point depression in °C.		0.114	0.226	0.337	0.447	0.506
The determined freezing point depression in °C.	0.104	0.198	0.381		0.728	0.890

In table 138 a comparison is made between the values of phenol found by other authors, and our own values.

Tabel 138.

Author	The concentration in %	The freezing point depression	The freezing point depression we find according to fig. 29
Landolt-Börnstein 1923	0.491	0.101	0.102
» »	1.153	0.228	0.227
» »	2.854	0.524	0.531
» »	3.7785	0.676	0.690
» »	4.607	0.843	0.828
Rosenthaler	2.95	0.56	0.548
Own result	2.8		0.520

Table 137 shows that there is a great difference between the values we find in the case of aqueous solutions of phenol when using the two methods of determination. As, however, it is seen in table 138 that there is good agreement between the values of *Landolt-Börnstein*'s tables and our freezing point depressions, the explanation must be that it is the vapour pressure determinations which have failed in the present case. This is probably due to the fact that phenol itself is volatile at the temperature at which the determinations of the vapour pressure of the aqueous solutions are made.

Phenosalylum.

Vapour pressure and freezing point determinations were made of the following solutions of phenosalyl. Phenosalyl is a solution containing 36 % phenol, 16 % citric acid, 5 % lactic acid, 4 % salicylic acid, 0.4 % menthol, 0.1 % oil of eucalyptus, 24 % glycerin, 10.5 % alcohol (90 per cent), and 4 % of water. The results are shown in table 139, and in the case of the vapour pressure determinations they are given in the corresponding freezing point depressions.

Table 139.

The concentration of phenosalyl grammes/1000 millilitres	10.00	20.00	30.00	40.00	50.00
Vapour pressure determination given in the corresponding freezing point depression in ^{0}C.	0.076	0.146	0.213		
The determined freezing point depression in ^{0}C.	0.172	0.335	0.493	0.648	0.806

As to the great difference between the results of the vapour pressure determinations and the freezing point determinations, the explanation must be the same as proposed in the case of phenol (p. 141). The freezing point determinations must be correct, as was the case with phenol. Evidently the vapour pressure determinations have failed, because phenosalyl itself is volatile at the temperature at which the vapour pressure determinations are made.

We have found no values in literature with which to compare our results.

Strychnini nitras.

Vapour pressure determinations were made of the following solutions of strychnine nitrate. In table 140 the results are given in the corresponding freezing point depressions.

Table 140.

The concentration of strychnine nitrate grammes/1000 millilitres	5.00	10.00
The corresponding freezing point depression in ^{0}C.	0.035	0.068

There is some disagreement between *Schou's* statement that a 1 % solution of strychnine nitrate should correspond to a 0.12 % solution of sodium chloride, which gives a freezing point depression of 0.074^0, and our result, which according to fig. 29 is 0.068^0.

On the other hand there is good agreement with *Ph. Norv.*, stating that 0.78 % of sodium chloride must be added to a 1 % solution of strychnine nitrate to obtain isoosmosis; we find the same value.

In fig. 29 the values of tables 129, 130, 132, 133, 134, 135, 137, 139, and 140 have been marked in the same manner as the values in fig. 6.

Fig. 29

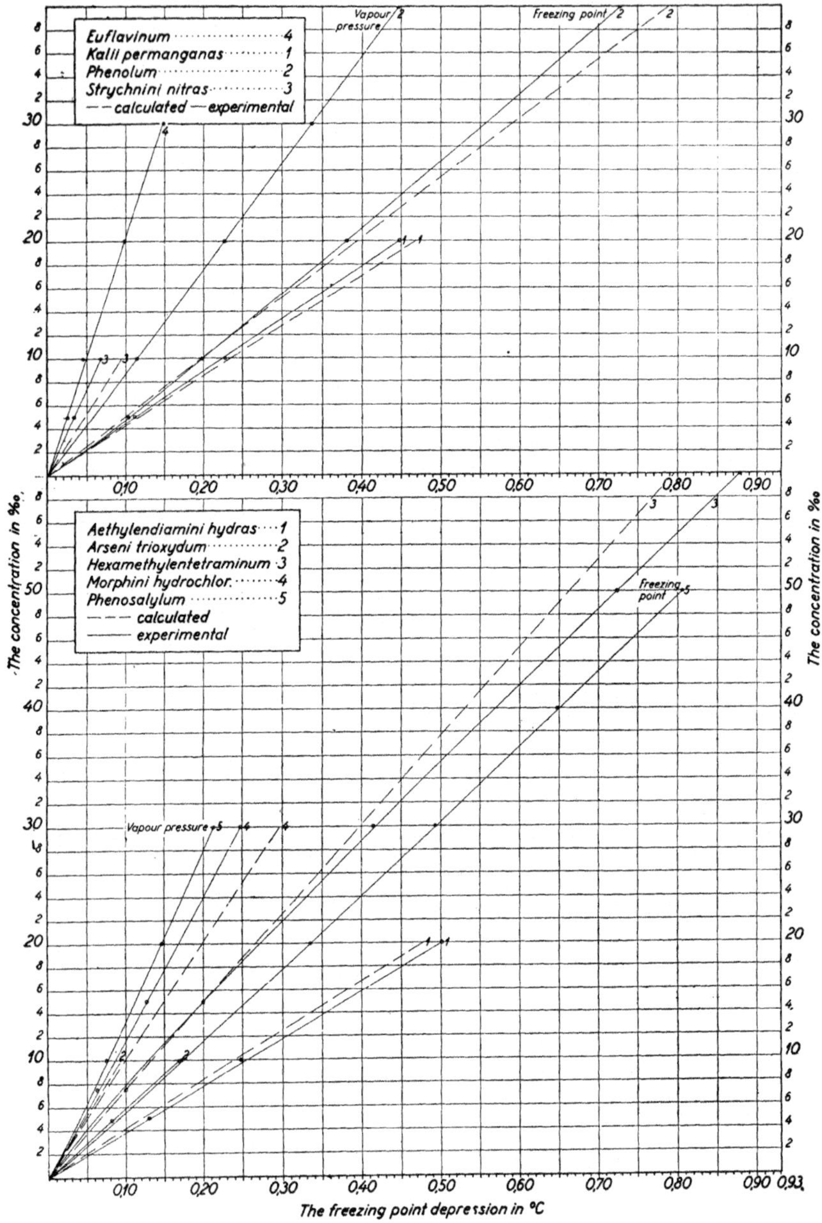
Euflavinum 4
Kalii permanganas 1
Phenolum 2
Strychnini nitras 3
calculated
experimental
Vapour pressure
Freezing point
Aethylendiamini hydras 1
Arseni trioxydum 2
Hexamethylentetraminum 3
Morphini hydrochlor. 4
Phenosalylum 5
calculated
experimental
Freezing point
Vapour pressure
The concentration in ‰
The freezing point depression in °C

Alcohol absolutus.

Besides the results of determinations already mentioned we have made some freezing point determinations of mixtures of ethyl alcohol and water, and the results of these determinations are given below, in table 141 and in fig. 30. These results have not been mentioned before, but that is due to the fact that in the case of ethyl alcohol we have made determinations within a much greater freezing point depression interval than in the case of the other substances.

Table 141.

The concentration of ethyl alcohol grammes/1000 millilitres	14.61	26.18	52.22	80.21
The determined freezing point depression in °C.	0.590	1.063	2.117	3.356

Fig. 30

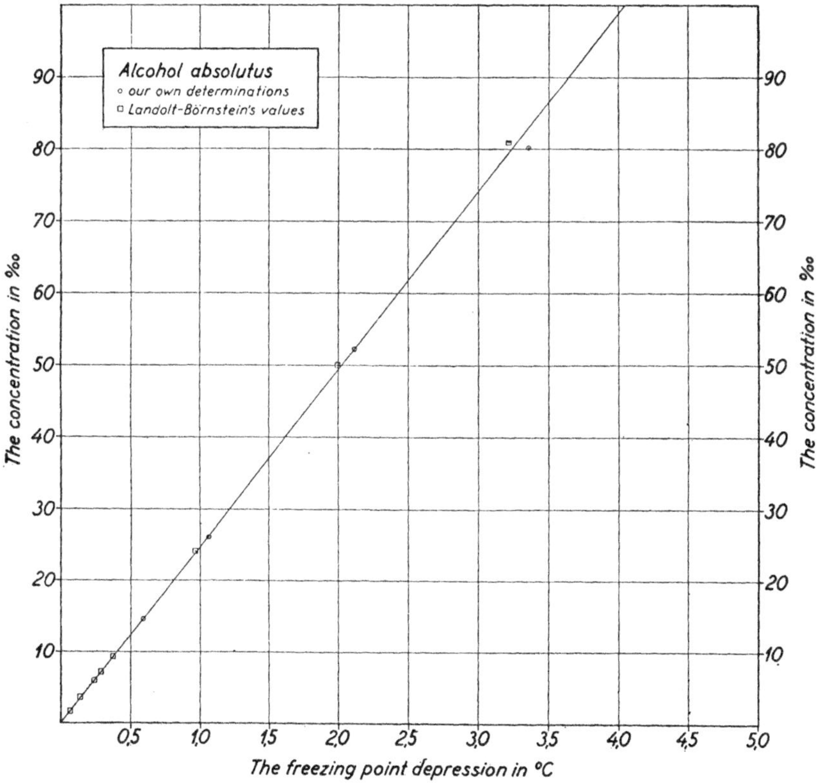

The values in table 141 have been marked in fig. 30 together with the values from *Landolt-Börnstein*. It will be seen from fig. 30 that there is good agreement between these values and our own, and that all the values practically lie on the straight line that is the calculated curve of ethyl alcohol.

As a proposal for the Danish pharmacopoeia the curves have been drawn on the basis of the determinations the results of which are given in figures 31—38. Fig. 39 shows the curves of some substances which are non-official in Denmark. These curves have only been drawn in the interval between the freezing point depression of 0° to 0.52°, which latter value is that of the isoosmotic solution. In these figures we have also drawn the mirrored sodium chloride curve, by means of which it is easy to find out how much sodium chloride must be added to a hypotonic solution of a substance in order to obtain isoosmosis. As to the method of reading the values from the drawing, we refer to fig. 3 of the present treatise.

While figures 31, 32, 33, 34, 35, 36, 37, and 39 only treat of substances which are applied internally, the substances for external application have been collected in fig. 38.

Fig. 31

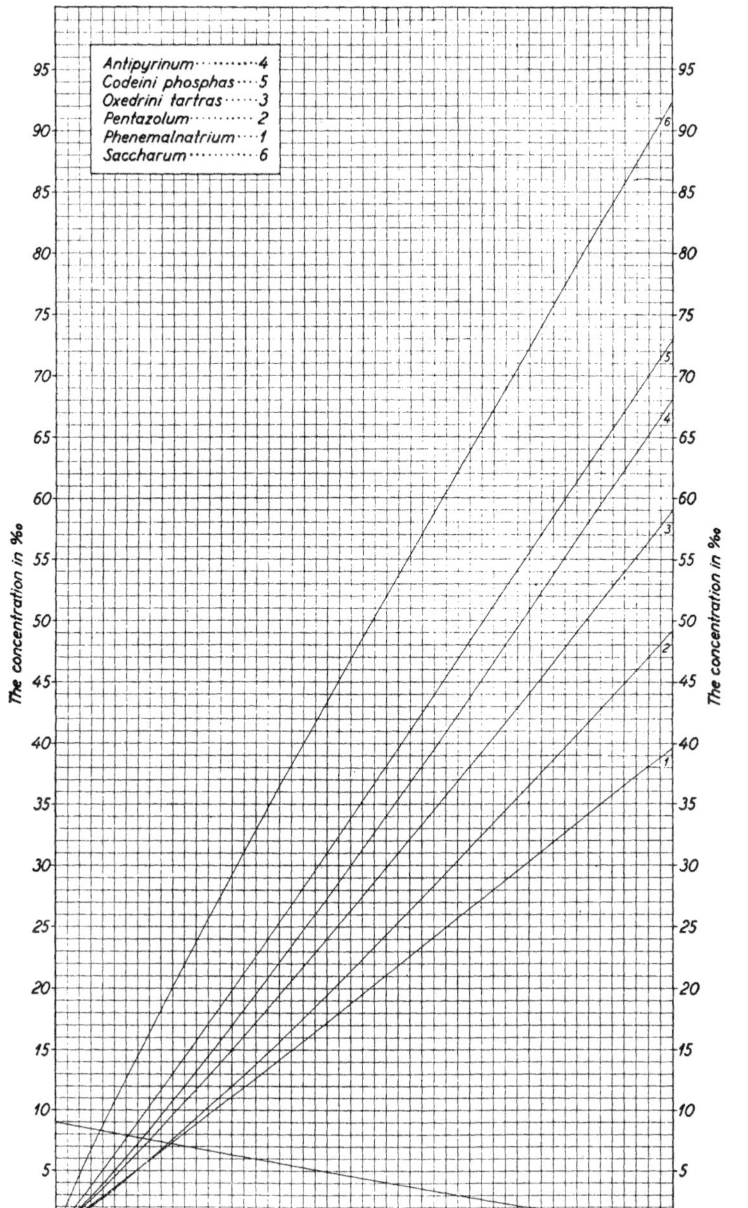

Antipyrinum 4
Codeini phosphas 5
Oxedrini tartras 3
Pentazolum 2
Phenemalnatrium 1
Saccharum 6
The concentration in ‰
The freezing point depression in °C
0,05 0,10 0,15 0,20 0,25 0,30 0,35 0,40 0,45 0,50 0,52
5 10 15 20 25 30 35 40 45 50 55 60 65 70 75 80 85 90 95

Fig. 32

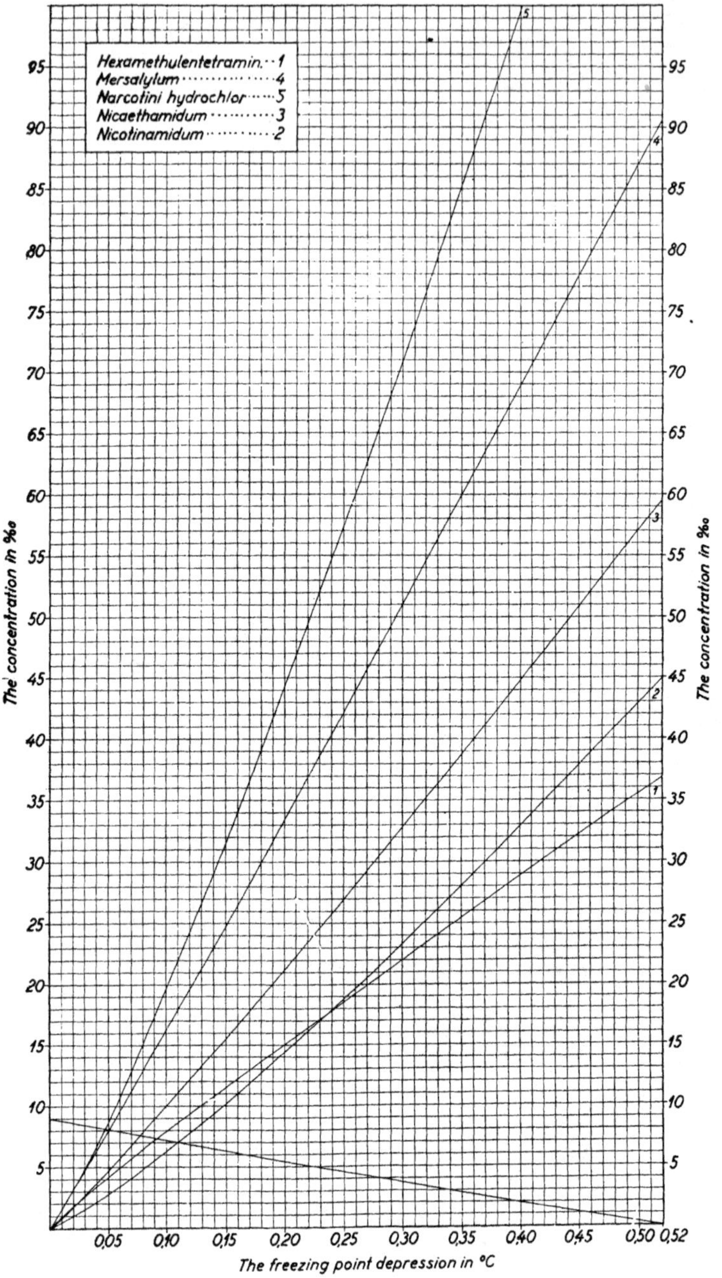

Hexamethulentetramin. 1
Mersalylum 4
Narcotini hydrochlor 5
Nicaethamidum 3
Nicotinamidum 2
The concentration in ‰
The freezing point depression in °C
0,05 0,10 0,15 0,20 0,25 0,30 0,35 0,40 0,45 0,50 0,52
5 10 15 20 25 30 35 40 45 50 55 60 65 70 75 80 85 90 95

Fig. 33

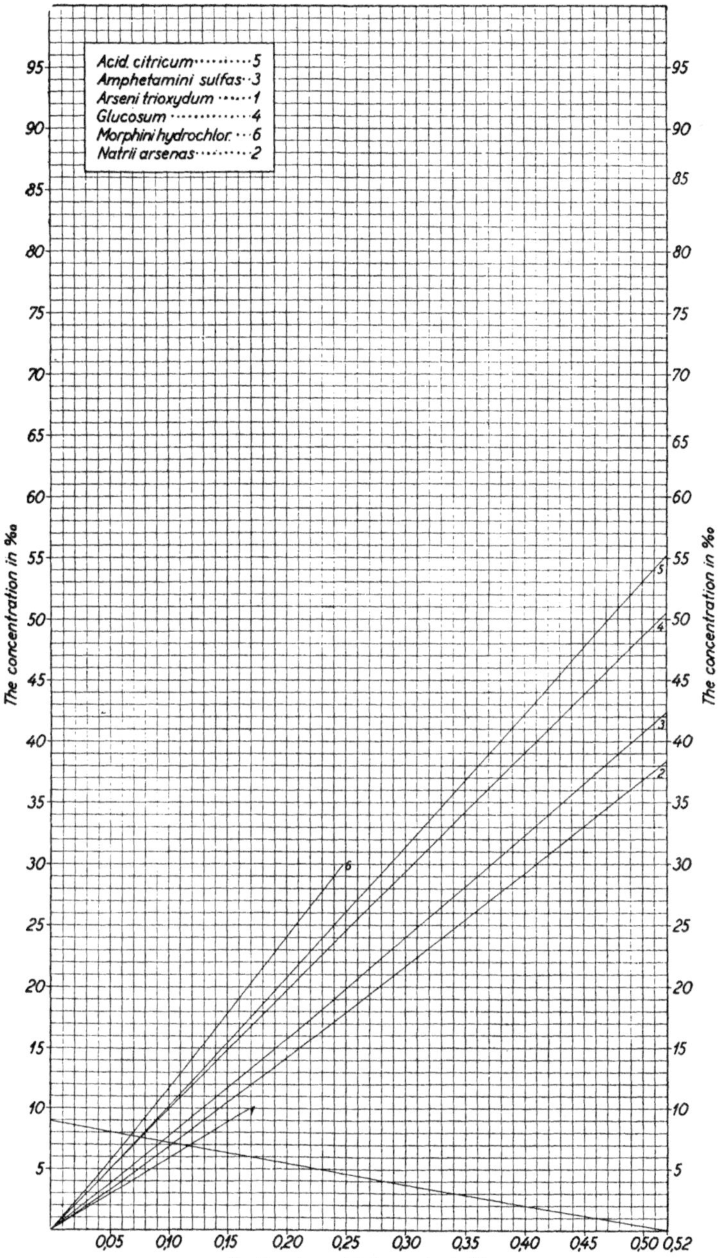

Acid. citricum ········ 5
Amphetamini sulfas ·· 3
Arseni trioxydum ····· 1
Glucosum ············· 4
Morphini hydrochlor. ··· 6
Natrii arsenas ········ 2
The concentration in ‰
The freezing point depression in °C
0,05
0,10
0,15
0,20
0,25
0,30
0,35
0,40
0,45
0,50
0,52

Fig.34

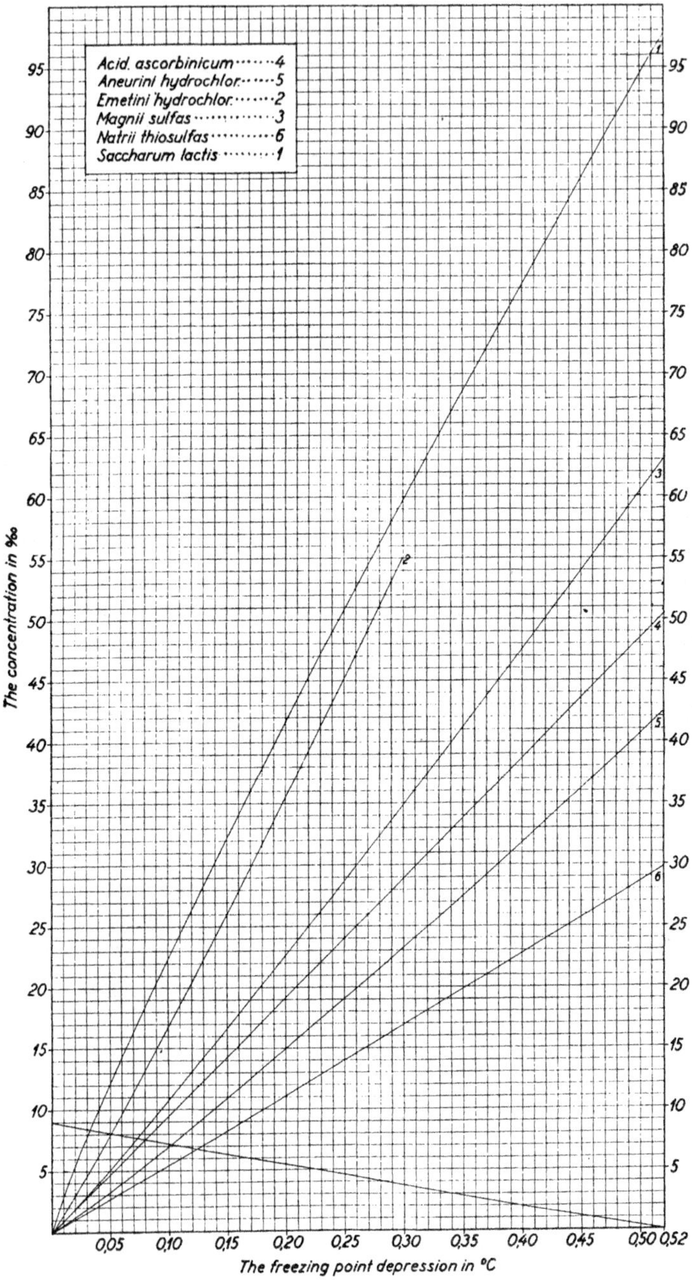
Acid. ascorbinicum 4
Aneurini hydrochlor. 5
Emetini hydrochlor. 2
Magnii sulfas 3
Natrii thiosulfas 6
Saccharum lactis 1
The concentration in ‰
The freezing point depression in °C
0,05 0,10 0,15 0,20 0,25 0,30 0,35 0,40 0,45 0,50 0,52
5 10 15 20 25 30 35 40 45 50 55 60 65 70 75 80 85 90 95

Fig.35

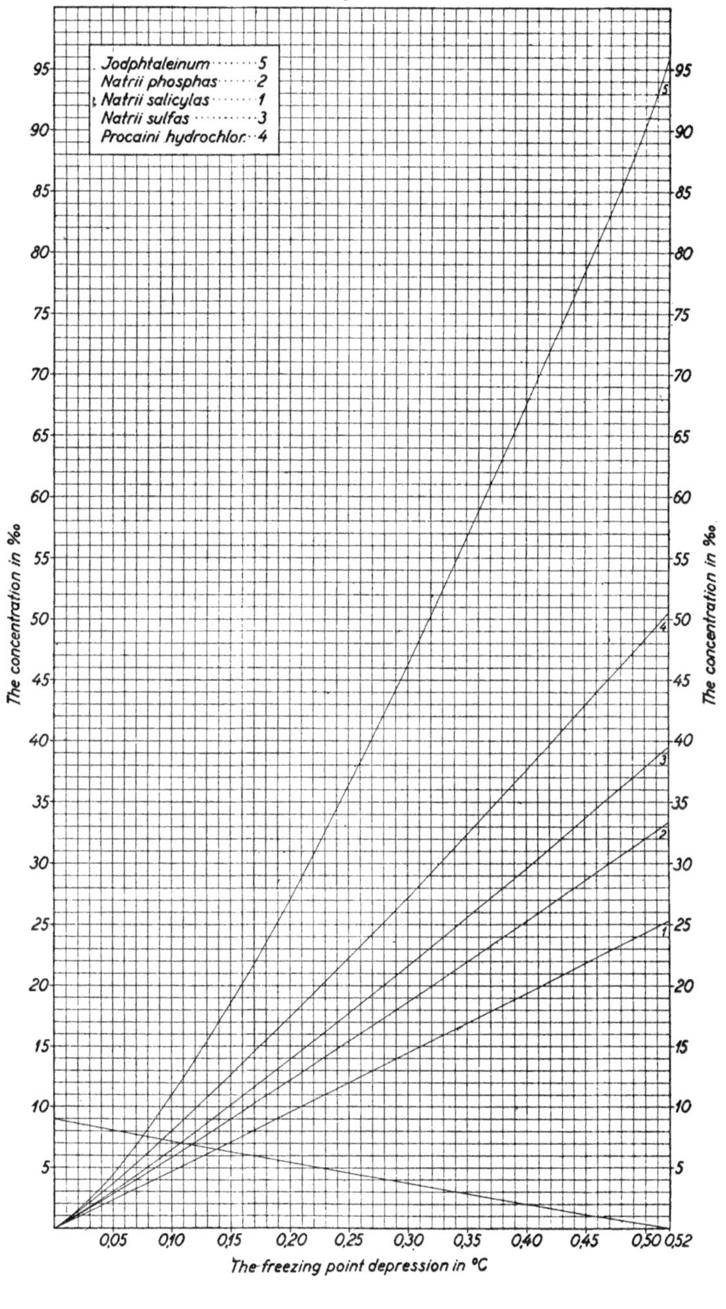

Jodphtaleinum ······· 5
Natrii phosphas ······ 2
Natrii salicylas ······· 1
Natrii sulfas ········· 3
Procaini hydrochlor. ·· 4
The concentration in ‰
The freezing point depression in °C
0,05 0,10 0,15 0,20 0,25 0,30 0,35 0,40 0,45 0,50 0,52
5 10 15 20 25 30 35 40 45 50 55 60 65 70 75 80 85 90 95

Fig. 36

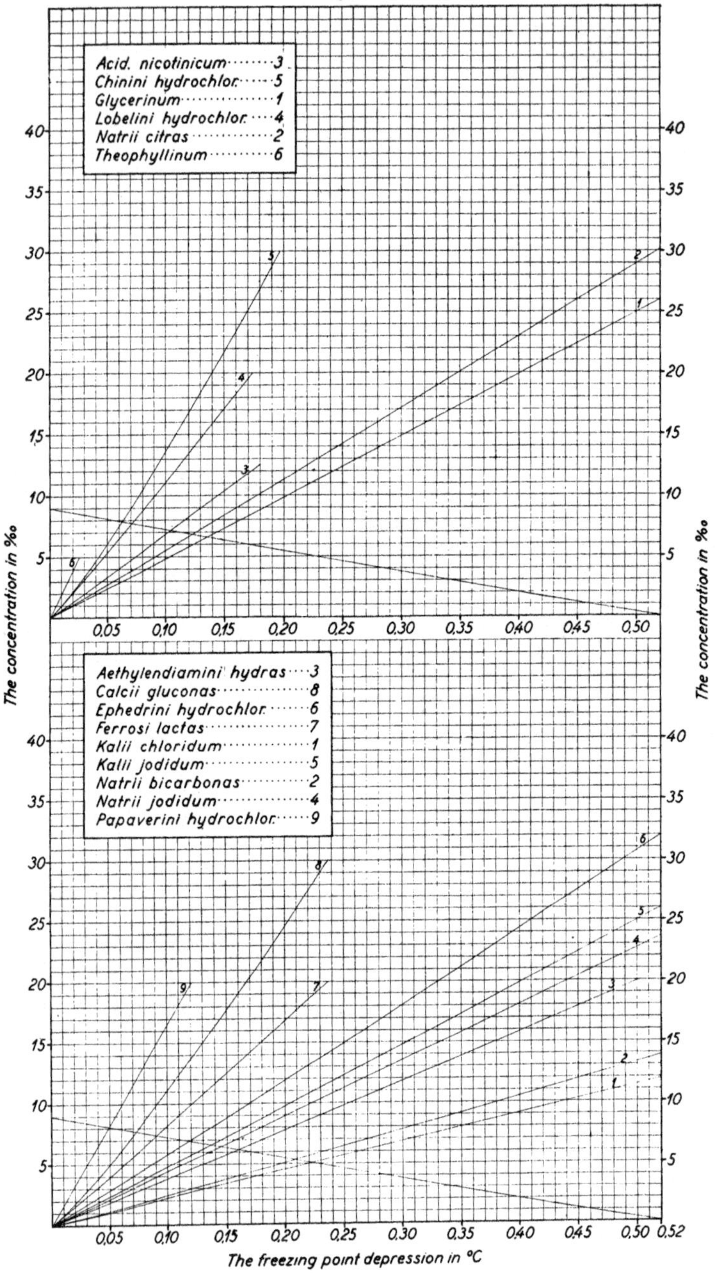
Acid. nicotinicum 3
Chinini hydrochlor. 5
Glycerinum 1
Lobelini hydrochlor. 4
Natrii citras 2
Theophyllinum 6
Aethylendiamini hydras ... 3
Calcii gluconas 8
Ephedrini hydrochlor. 6
Ferrosi lactas 7
Kalii chloridum 1
Kalii jodidum 5
Natrii bicarbonas 2
Natrii jodidum 4
Papaverini hydrochlor. ... 9
The concentration in ‰
The freezing point depression in °C

Fig. 37

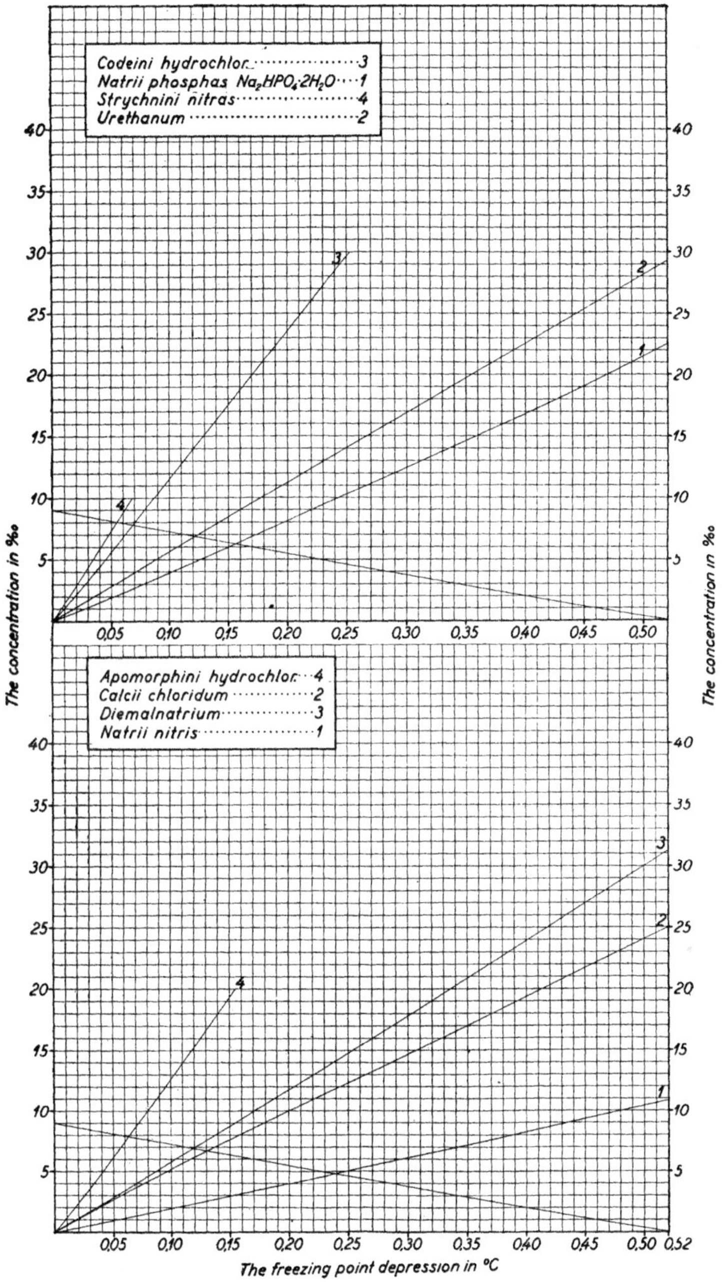

Codeini hydrochlor. ... 3
Natrii phosphas $Na_2HPO_4 \cdot 2H_2O$ ... 1
Strychnini nitras ... 4
Urethanum ... 2
Apomorphini hydrochlor. ... 4
Calcii chloridum ... 2
Diemalnatrium ... 3
Natrii nitris ... 1
The concentration in ‰
The freezing point depression in °C

Fig. 38

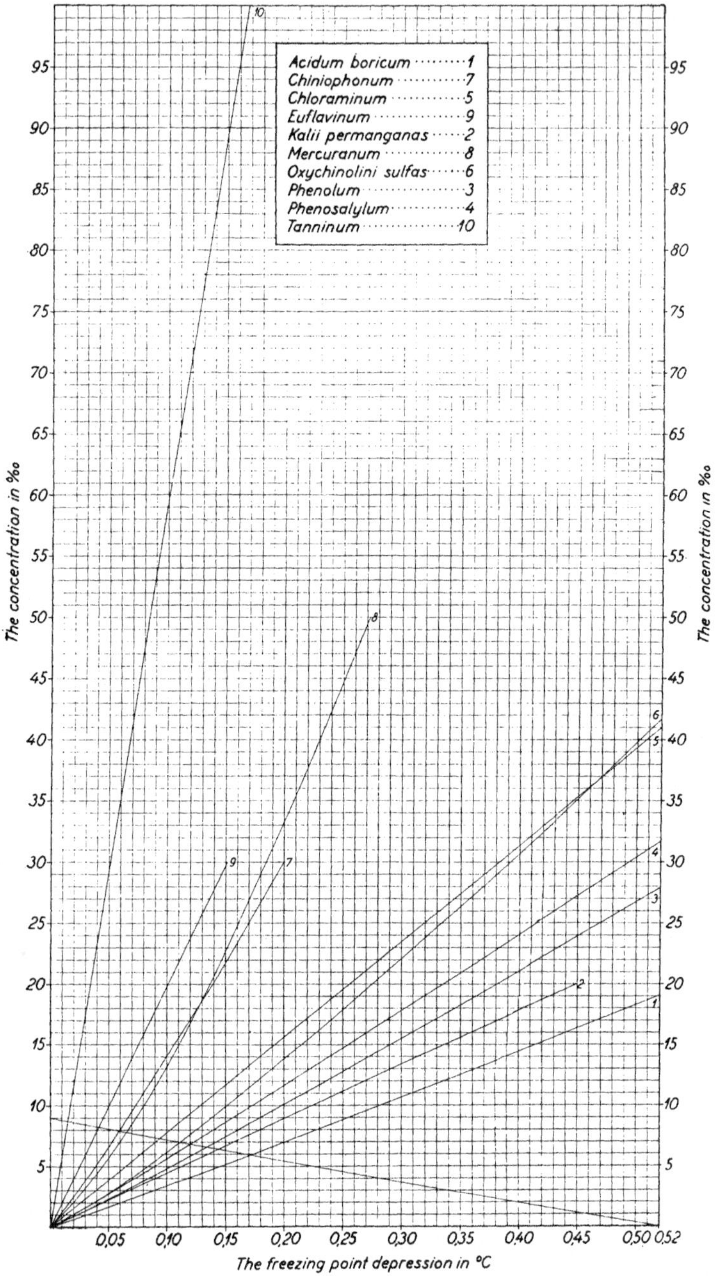
Acidum boricum 1
Chiniophonum 7
Chloraminum 5
Euflavinum 9
Kalii permanganas 2
Mercuranum 8
Oxychinolini sulfas 6
Phenolum 3
Phenosalylum 4
Tanninum 10
The concentration in ‰
The freezing point depression in °C
0,05 0,10 0,15 0,20 0,25 0,30 0,35 0,40 0,45 0,50 0,52
5 10 15 20 25 30 35 40 45 50 55 60 65 70 75 80 85 90 95

Fig. 39

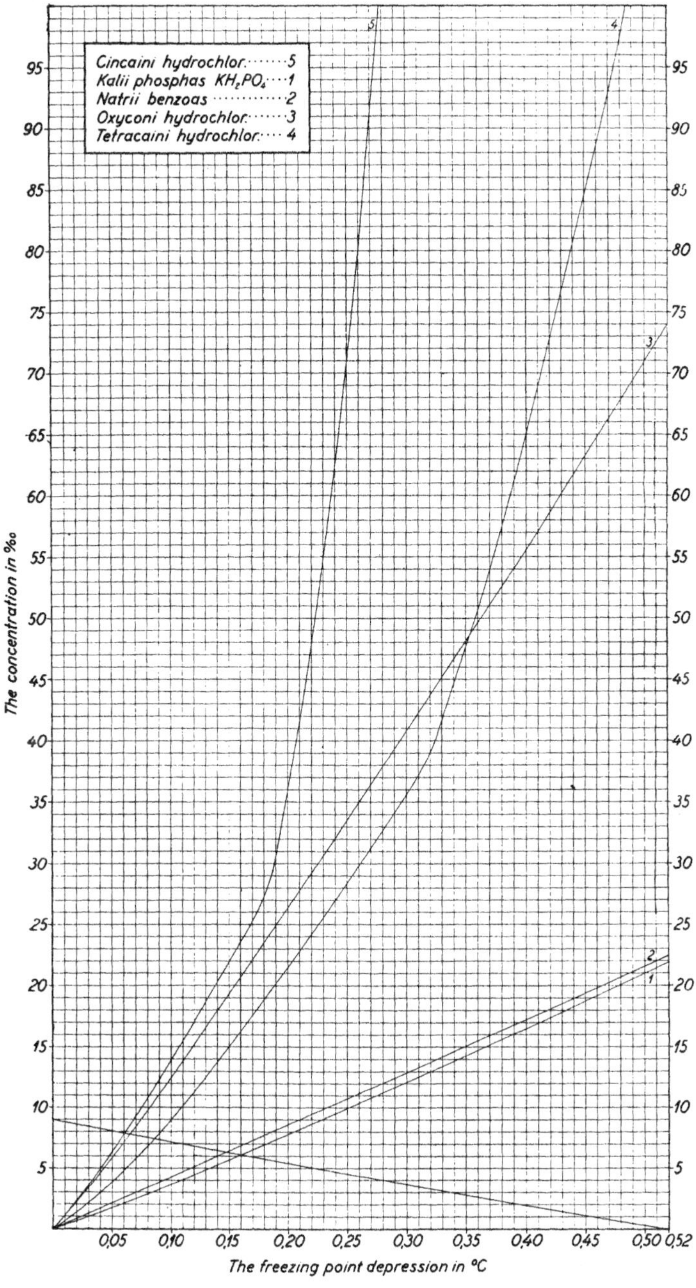
Cincaini hydrochlor. 5
Kalii phosphas KH_2PO_4 1
Natrii benzoas 2
Oxyconi hydrochlor. 3
Tetracaini hydrochlor. 4
The concentration in ‰
The freezing point depression in °C
0,05 0,10 0,15 0,20 0,25 0,30 0,35 0,40 0,45 0,50 0,52
5 10 15 20 25 30 35 40 45 50 55 60 65 70 75 80 85 90 95

4. *Activity relations.*

In figures 21—29 both the calculated and the experimentally found freezing point depressions have been marked in pairs thus giving a graphic impression of the activity relations.

The *calculated* values all form straight lines. In the logarithmic system they are parallel, and form an angle of 45° with the ordinate.

The *experimental* values in most cases also form straight lines in the logarithmic system, but the lines are not parallel, the angle formed with the ordinate being in some cases greater, and in some smaller than 45°, and in some cases = 45°.

The substances which do not form straight lines in the logarithmic system are amethocaine (fig. 26) and cinchocaine (fig. 26) both of which show a straightlined course from the zero-point of the system of coordinates. This straight line is interrupted at a certain concentration (amethocaine: 3.8 %, cinchocaine: 2.7 %), from which points the curves still continue to be straight, but at a steeper angle. The angles that these two substances at first form with the ordinate in the logarithmic system amount to 51.9° and 47.8° respectively, after the bend, however, they amount to 65.6° and 70.9° respectively. In the arithmetical system these two substances show a remarkably steep course of the curve; thus there is not much difference between the freezing point depressions caused by solutions of 5 % and 10 % (amethocaine 5 % = 0.358°, 10 % = 0.485°, cinchocaine 5 % = 0.223°, 10 % = 0.278°). Alypine hydrochloride, which is described in the first part of this paper, shows similar conditions.

When the experimental curves in the logarithmic system are straight and form angles of 45° with the ordinate, the activity coefficients of the substances will prove to be constant, irrespective of the concentration. These curves will prove to be straight also in the arithmetical system. Substances representative of this group are sodium benzoate and urethane.

When the experimental curves in the logarithmic system are straight and form angles of less than 45° with the ordinate, the activity coefficients of the substances will prove to decrease, when the concentration increases. In the arithmetical system these curves will form parabolic figures, the ordinate being their axis. By far the greater number of substances belong to this group, of which the following substances may be mentioned: magnesium sulphate, sodium sulphate, nicotinamide, and leptazole.

When the experimental curves in the logarithmic system are straight and form angles of more than 45° with the ordinate, the activity coefficients of the substances will increase when the concentrations increase. In the arithmetical system these curves will form parabolic figures, the abscissa being their axis. The following substances may be mentioned as representative of this group: calcium chloride, hexamine, sucrose, and lactose.

By means of the calculated and the experimental curves shown in figures 21—29 the activity coefficients have been found of such solutions of the substances as give a freezing point depression of 0.186°, 0.52°, and 0.93°, in so far as the solubility of the substances has made it possible to make the necessary concentrations. The three mentioned freezing point depressions are brought about in a non-electrolyte of 0.1, 0.28, and 0.5 molar solutions respectively. The results are given in table 142.

Table 142.

The name of the substance	Freezing point depression:		
	0.186 °	0.52 °	0.93 °
	The activity coefficient		
Acidum ascorbinicum	0.984	0.977	0.973
Acidum boricum	0.962	0.915	0.890
Acidum citricum	1.088	1.053	
Acidum nicotinicum	0.952		
Aethylendiamini hydras	1.086	1.050	
Amphetamini sulfas	0.833	0.812	0.800
Aneurini hydrachloridum	1.193	1.100	1.049
Antipyrinum	0.870	0.772	
Apomorphini hydrochloridum	0.656		
Calcii chloridum	0.763	0.808	0.835
Calcii gluconas	0.660		
Chinini hydrochloridum	0.742		
Cincaini hydrochloridum	0.698	0.437	0.295
Codeini hydrochloridum	0.855		
Codeini phosphas	0.851	0.812	
Diemalnatrium	0.941	0.921	0.912
Emetini hydrochloridum	0.850		
Ephedrini hydrochloridum	0.950	0.882	0.866
Ferrosi lactas	0.612		
Glucosum (anhydricum)	0.980	0.997	1.000
Glycerinum	1.005	0.990	0.983
Hexamethylentetraminum	1.000	1.071	1.108
Jodphtaleinum	1.081	0.846	
Kalii chloridum	0.883	0.881	0.877
Kalii jodidum	0.917	0.894	0.883
Kalii permanganas	0.950	0.950	
Kalii phosphas KH_2PO_4	0.941	0.881	0.842
Lobelini hydrochloridum	0.876		
Magnii sulfas	0.608	0.569	0.548

Table 142 (continued).

The name of the substance	Freezing point depression:		
	0.186°	0.52°	0.93°
	The activity coefficient		
Mercuranum	0.828		
Mersalylum	0.818	0.782	
Morphini hydrochloridum	0.849		
Narcotini hydrochloridum	0.577		
Natrii arsenas $Na_2HAsO_4 \cdot 7H_2O$	0.789	0.755	0.743
Natrii bicarbonas	0.874	0.842	0.827
Natrii citras $C_6H_5O_7Na_3 \cdot 2H_2O$	0.710	0.690	0.675
Natrii jodidum	0.907	0.884	0.853
Natrii nitris	0.936	0.893	0.858
Natrii phosphas $Na_2HPO_4 \cdot 7H_2O$	0.801	0.756	0.739
Natrii phosphas $Na_2HPO_4 \cdot 2H_2O$	0.796	0.758	0.734
Natrii salicylas	0.893	0.885	0.879
Natrii sulfas	0.839	0.761	0.721
Natrii thiosulfas	0.801	0.781	0.767
Nicaethamidum	0.913	0.835	
Nicotinamidum	0.917	0.758	0.676
Oxedrini tartras	0.842	0.779	
Oxyconi hydrochloridum	0.840	0.770	
Papaverini hydrochloridum	0.618		
Pentazolum	0.902	0.785	0.729
Phenemalnatrium	0.907	0.894	0.882
Phenolum	1.000	0.946	
Procaini hydrochloridum	0.855	0.781	0.731
Saccharum	0.955	1.036	
Saccharum lactis	0.918	1.033	
Tetracaini hydrochloridum	0.780	0.621	0.451
Urethanum	0.844	0.848	0.848

5. *Discussion.*

In order to obtain isoosmotic solutions for parenteral injection and solutions for application to injured tissue, we have in the preceding pages described the osmotic conditions, expressed by means of the freezing point depressions of aqueous solutions of 67 different substances, most of which are official.

The freezing point depressions have been found partly through calculation, partly experimentally by means of determinations of the freezing point of the solution itself, in relation to distilled water, or by means of determinations of the vapour pressure of the solution, in relation to sodium chloride solutions of a known concentration. In the case of the determination of the freezing point depression, correction has been made for the amount of disengaged ice.

The calculation of the freezing point depression is based on the molar freezing point depression of 1.86°. The number of ions into which a substance is ionised, has been taken into consideration, but not contingent activity factors, as they are only available in the case of a limited number of the substances we have examined.

In figures 21—29 the curves have been drawn partly on the basis of the calculated, partly on the experimentally found values. In this manner we have obtained graphically an insight into the activity relations of the substances. They may be divided into several groups:

a. Most of the substances show a smaller experimental freezing point depression than had been calculated, corresponding to an activity coefficient smaller than 1. In the case of the majority of the substances belonging to this group, the activity coefficient will decrease when the concentration increases; in the case of a small number of substances of this group the activity coefficient is constant within the interval in question.

b. A few substances, as sucrose and glycerin, show almost the same freezing point depression by experimental determination and by calculation, corresponding to an activity coefficient aqual to 1.

c. Some substances show a greater freezing point depression by experimental determination than by calculation, corresponding to an activity coefficient greater than 1.

d. Finally some substances show an activity coefficient which in the lower concentrations is greater than 1, whereas in the higher concentrations it is smaller than 1, and at the concentration where the calculated and the experimental curves intersect, the coefficient is equal to 1. Other substances, however, show a direct contrary course, the activity coefficients in the lower concentrations being smaller than 1, in the higher concentrations greater than 1.

The activity relations of the substances are also shown in table 142, where the activity coefficients of solutions with freezing point depressions of 0.186°, 0.52°, and 0.93° have been given, in so far as the solubility of the substances has made it possible to produce the necessary concentrations.

In table 143 a comparison is made between our activity coefficients and those of the »*International Critical Tables*« (1929). The accordance between the two sets of values is not complete, which may be due to the fact that two different methods of determination have been used, the values of the above mentioned tables being based on determinations of the freezing point depressions, whereas our values, as mentioned, are based on vapour pressure determinations. In changing the values of our vapour pressure determinations into freezing point values we have employed a sodium chloride curve, which has been corrected because of the disengaged ice. If this correction is not made, an activity coefficient is arrived at that is about 5 % higher, and that corresponds with the activity coefficients stated in the »*International Critical Tables*».

Table 143.

The activity coefficient of 0.1 molar solutions.

The name of the substance	International Critical Tables	Own results
Calcii chloridum	0.867	0.822
Kalii chloridum	0.929	0.882
Kalii jodidum	0.953	0.900
Kalii nitras	0.892	0.876
Kalii phosphas (KH_2PO_4)	0.899	0.891
Magnii sulfas	0.606	0.558
Natrii chloridum	0.936	0.928
Natrii sulfas	0.779	0.757
Natrii phosphas ($Na_2HPO_4 \cdot 2H_2O$)	0.779	0.740

It has been shown that the freezing point depression of a solution of several different substances cannot always be found simply by adding the freezing point depressions of each single substance. This is, for instance, the case when acids and bases are neutralized, and occurs in the following preparations: sol. acid, ascorbin. pro injectione, and sol. ergometrini pro injectione, where the acid in both cases reacts with the solution of sodium bicarbonate, at the same time generating carbon dioxide. Here the freezing point depressions of the prepared solutions are smaller than the sums of the freezing point depressions of the components. Thus when boric acid is neutralized with sodium hydroxide the solution of sodium borate thus made gives a smaller freezing point depression than the sum of the freezing point depressions of boric acid and sodium hydroxide. In the latter case the effect is not due to volatile compounds, but must be ascribed to the transformation of orthoborate into tetraborate.

Some mixtures of glycerin and water also show a deviating course of the curve because mixtures of low glycerin content and mixtures of low water content have the same freezing point depressions as shown in table 144 and figure 40, the values of which have been taken from the »*Handbook of Chemistry and Physics*« 1936—37.

Table 144.

The concentration of glycerin in %	The corresponding freezing point depression in °C
10	+ 1.6
20	+ 4.8
30	+ 9.5
40	+ 15.4
50	+ 23.0
60	+ 34.7
70	+ 38.9
80	+ 20.3
90	+ 1.6
100	— 17.0

Fig. 40

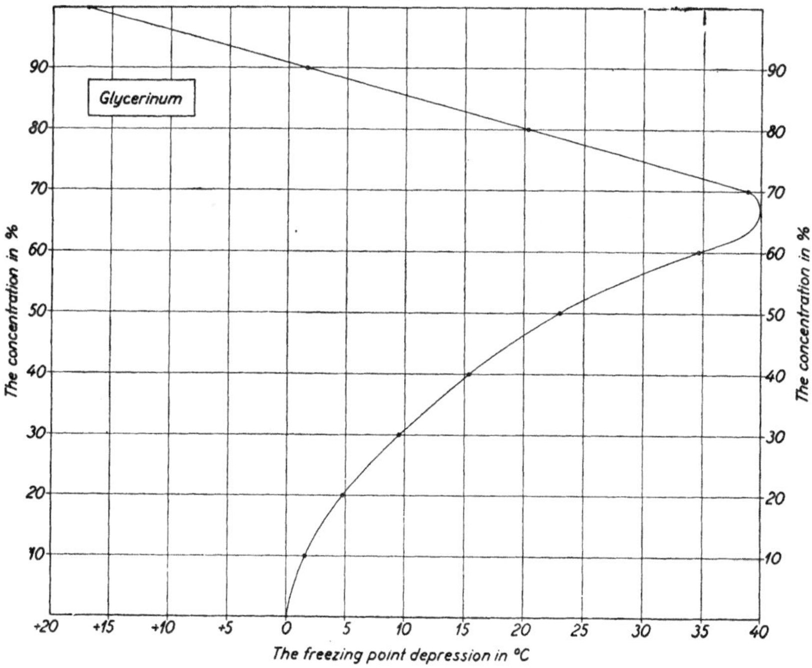

As a proposal for a future Danish pharmacopoeia the curves from 0^0 to 0.52^0 freezing point depression have been drawn on the basis of the experimental determinations, and are shown in figures 31—39. These figures, as well as the experimental curves in figures 21—29 have been drawn in the arithmetical system, as it is the easier system in which to work. First, however, the obtained results of the determinations have been marked in a system of coordinates, where the logarithm of the freezing point depression has been marked along the abscissa, and the logarithm of the concentration along the ordinate. The line connecting these points is in nearly all the examined substances a straight one, and can therefore be represented with very great accuracy. By calculating the equation, which is the expression of this line it is possible to transfer the latter, point by point, into the arithmetical system of coordinates, where, as a rule, the curves show a more or less arched course, and so require a considerably greater number of marked points than the straight line needs in order to be drawn with reasonable accuracy.

6. Control of the official solutions for injection.

Finally we have determined the vapour pressure of most of the solutions for injection that are described in the Pharmacopoea Danica, Dispensatorium Danicum, and in the DAK. The results are given in table 145.

Table 145.

The name of the solution for injection	The present freezing point depression	Is the composition to be altered
Injectabile amphetamini DAK	slightly hyperosmotic (0.61^0)	No
» aneurini 2.5 % DAK	isoosmotic	No
» aneurini 1 % DAK	isoosmotic	No
» ferrosi lactatis DAK	slightly hyperosmotic (0.57^0)	No
» lactoflavini DAK	strongly hyperosmotic (1.51^0)	No
» nicotinamidi DAK	slightly hyperosmotic (0.57^0)	No
» sulfathiazoli DAK	strongly hyperosmotic (cannot be determined)	
Liquor ad solut. procain. D.D.	see solventium ad procainum	
Liquor natrii chloridi phenolatus D.D.	slightly hyperosmotic	Yes, into 0.75 % of sodium chloride.
Solutio acid ascorbin. pro inj. D.D.	slightly hyperosmotic (0.42^0)	Yes, add 0.20 % of sodium chloride.
Solutio adrenalini hydrochlor. pro inj. Ph. Dan.	isoosmotic (0.53^0)	No

Table 145 (continued).

The name of the solution for injection	The present freezing point depression	Is the composition to be altered
Solutio apomorphini hydrochlor. pro inj. Ph. Dan.	hypoosmotic	Yes, add 0.70 % of sodium chloride.
Solutio arseni trioxyd. pro inj. Ph. Dan.	isoosmotic (0.52^0)	No
Solutio atropini sulfat. pro inj. D.D.	isoosmotic (0.52^0)	No
Solutio calcii chloridi pro inj. intraven. D.D.	strongly hyperosmotic (2.28^0)	No
Solutio calcii gluconat. pro inj. D D.	hyperosmotic (0.65^0)	No
Solutio chinini hydrochlor. pro inj. D.D.	strongly hyperosmotic (1.97^0)	No
Solutio coffeini pro inj. D.D.	strongly hyperosmotic (5.3^0)	No
Solutio diemalnatrii pro inj. D.D.	strongly hyperosmotic (5.3^0)	No
Solutio emetini hydrochlor. pro inj. D.D.	slightly hypoosmotic	Yes, into 0.45 % of sodium chloride.
Solutio ephedrini hydrochlor. pro inj. D.D.	hyperosmotic (0.80^0)	No
Sol. ergometrini pro inj. D.D.	isoosmotic (0.52^0)	No
Sol. glucosi pro inj. intraven. D.D.	hyperosmotic (1.03^0)	No
Sol. histamini hydrochlor. pro inj. D.D.	isoosmotic (0.52^0)	No
Sol. hypnopheni pro inj. Ph. Dan.	strongly hyperosmotic (cannot be determined)	No
Sol. invertosi pro inj. D.D.	strongly hyperosmotic (9^0)	No
Sol. lobelini hydrochlor. pro inj. D.D.	isoosmotic (0.52^0)	No
Sol. magnii sulfat. pro inj. D.D.	strongly hyperosmotic (1.54^0)	No
Sol. mersalyli pro inj. D.D.	slightly hyperosmotic (0.62^0)	No
Sol. methylthionini chlorid. pro inj. intraven. D.D.	slightly hyperosmotic (0.62^0)	Yes, into 3.5 % of Na_2SO_4
Sol. morphini citrat. fort. DAK.	isoosmotic (0.52^0)	No
Sol. morphini citrat mitior DAK.	isoosmotic (0.52^0)	No
Sol. morphini hydrochlor. pro inj. Ph. Dan.	strongly hyperosmotic (cannot be determined)	No
Sol. natrii auri chlorid. pro inj. intraven. D.D.	isoosmotic (0.52^0)	No
Sol. natrii bicarbon. isotonica Ph. Dan.	slightly hypoosmotic	Yes, into 1.4 % of $NaHCO_3$
Sol. natrii chlorid. pro inj. Ph. Dan.	isoosmotic (0.52^0)	No
Sol. natrii citrat. ad transfusion. D.D.	slightly hypoosmotic	Yes, into 3.0 % of sodium citrate

Table 145 (continued).

The name of the solution for injection	The present freezing point depression	Is the composition to be altered
Sol. natrii sulfat. pro inj. intraven. D.D.	strongly hyperosmotic (2.37°)	No
Sol. natrii thiosulfat. pro inj. intraven. D.D.	strongly hyperosmotic (2.60°)	No
Solutio nicaethamidi pro inj. D.D.	strongly hyperosmotic (1.94°)	No
Sol. opiopapaverini comp. pro inj. D.D.	strongly hyperosmotic (4.8°)	No
Sol. oxedrini pro inj. D.D.	hyperosmotic (0.63°)	No
Sol. pentazoli pro inj. D. D.	hyperosmotic (0.94°)	No
Sol. phenemalnatrii pro inj. D.D.	strongly hyperosmotic (cannot be determined)	No
Sol. pilocarpini hydrochlor. pro inj. D.D.	isoosmotic (0.52°)	No
Sol. procaini hydrochlor. dentalis 1 % D.D.	hyperosmotic	Yes, K_2SO_4 is left out, add only 0.65 % of NaCl.
Sol. procaini hydrochlor. dentalis 2 % D.D.	hyperosmotic	Yes, K_2SO is left out, add only 0.4 % of NaCl.
Sol. procaini hydrochlor. fortior pro inj. D.D.	hyperosmotic	Yes, K_2SO is left out, add only 0.6 % of NaCl.
Sol. procaini hydrochlor. pro inj. D.D.	hyperosmotic	Yes, K_2SO_4 is left out, add only 0.75 % of NaCl.
Sol. scopolamini hydrobromid. pro inj. D.D.	isoosmotic (0.52°)	No
Sol. scopolamini hydrobromid. c. tetrapono pro inj. D.D.	strongly hyperosmotic (4.5°)	No
Sol. g-strophanthini pro inj. intraven. D.D.	isoosmotic (0.52°)	No
Sol. strychnini nitrat. pro inj. D.D.	isoosmotic (0.52°)	No
Sol. tetraponi pro inj. Ph. Dan.	strongly hyperosmotic (4.6°)	No
Sol. theophylamini fort. pro inj. D.D.	strongly hyperosmotic (2.1°)	No
Sol. theophylamini pro inj. D.D.	hypoosmotic	Yes, add 0.40 % of NaCl.
Solventium ad procainum: Natrii chlorid. 9 grammes Acid. hydrochlor. dil. 0.3 grammes Aq. dest. steril. 990.7 grammes	isoosmotic (0.52°)	No

It will be seen from table 145 that most of the solutions for injection have such freezing point depressions that there is no reason for altering their composition. It must be noted, however, that the majority of the solutions are hyperosmotic, and that it is impossible to alter this condition towards isoosmosis unless the concentration is made weaker, and in most cases this is hardly practicable, in view of the therapeutic effect.

It is with a certain saticfaction that one notices that solutions as *injectabile amphetamini* and *injectabile nicotinamidi* are almost isotonic. It would be preferable if substances such as oxedrini tartras, pentazolum, and glucosum were also made as 5 % solutions for injection, as these 5 substances have this in common, that an aqueous solution of 5 % is almost isotonic.

It is proposed, in reference to table 145, to add 0.2 % of sodium chloride to sol. acid. ascorbin. pro inj., to add 0.7 % of sodium chloride to sol. apomorphin. hydrochlor. pro inj., and to increase the concentration of sodium chloride in sol. emetini hydrochlor. pro inj. from 0.25 % to 0.45 %. The present concentration of sol. natrii bicarbon. isotonica has been found by means of calculation, but according to the results of our own determinations it must be changed from 1.3 % to 1.4 %. Furthermore the concentration of sodium citrate in sol. natrii citrat. ad transfusionem ought to be changed from 2.5 % to 3.0 %.

All the official solutions of procaine are hypertonic. If potassium sulphate is to be left out of these preparations, it is proposed at the same time to regulate the concentration of sodium chloride, so that these concentrations become isotonic.

7. Control of the official solutions for local application to tissues.

When it was reported to the dispensary of Bispebjerg Hospital that the patients in the surgical division of the hospital complained of great pain, when larger parts of tissue were submitted to a direct treatment with an 0.1 % solution of chloramine, the immediate explanation was that the pain must be due to the strongly hypotonic solution. When 0.9 % of sodium chloride was added the pain and the complaints ceased altogether. That was the reason why we made determinations of the solutions that have been mentioned in table 146, and which are generally applied in the treatment of mucous membranes when the epithelium has been injured, and of tissues in which strongly anisotonic solutions cause pain.

It will be seen that most of the solutions examined in table 146 are more or less hypoosmotic, so they ought to have sodium chloride added to them, (in the case of the solution of silver nitrate, how-

Table 146.

The name of the solution:	The present freezing point depression:	Is the composition to be altered?
Aqua calcis chloratae D.D.	slightly hyperosmotic (0.56°)	No
Liquor Dakin D.D.	hyperosmotic (1.2°)	No
Solutio acidi borici Ph. Dan.	isoosmotic	No
Solutio argent. nitrat. profylact. D.D.	hypoosmotic (0.38°)	Yes, add 0.45 % of potassium nitrate.
Solutio chloramini 0.1 %	hypoosmotic (0.013°)	Yes, add 0.9 % of sodium chloride.
Solutio euflavini D.D.	isoosmotic	No
Solutio euflavini conc. D.D.	hypoosmotic (0.05°)	Yes, add 0.8 % of sodium chloride.
Solutio kalii permanganat D.D.	strongly hypoosmotic	Yes, add 0.9 % of sodium chloride.
Solutio nitrat. argent. fort. F.n.c.h.	hypoosmotic (0.38°)	Yes, add 0.45 % of potassium nitrate.
Solutio nitrat. argent. mit. F.n.c.h.	hypoosmotic (0.038°)	Yes, add 1.50 % of potassium nitrate.
Solutio phenoli Ph. Dan.	hypoosmotic (0.38°)	Yes, add 0.25 % of sodium chloride.
Solutio phenosalyli D.D.	hypoosmotic (0.175°)	Yes, add 0.60 % of sodium chloride.

ever, potassium nitrate must be added), so that isotonic solutions are obtained. Sol. euflavini D. D., however, has been made isotonic by adding sodium chloride.

8. Summary.

The aim of this work has been to procure a basis for obtaining isoosmotic solutions, not only for parenteral injection, but also for local treatment of tissues. For this purpose we have given an account of the osmotic conditions, expressed by means of the freezing point depressions of aqueous solutions of 67 of the more commonly used substances. In most of the cases we have determined the vapour pressure of the solutions in relation to the vapour pressure of known solutions of sodium chloride, by means of *Hill*'s thermoelectric method. Then the results have been changed into the corresponding freezing point depressions. It is only in cases where this has not been possible, that we have determined the freezing point depression directly by means of *Beckmann*'s thermometer, and then we have corrected the results due to the amount of disengaged ice. The results have been shown graphically, first in a system where the ordinate is the logarithm of the concentration, and the abscissa is the logarithm of the freezing point depression. The straight line thus formed has then been moved into a corresponding arithmetical system, where the ordinate is the concentration, and the abscissa the freezing point depression and here the result is either a straight line, or a more or less arched curve.

In the case of each substance the results have been revised and compared with the results found by other authors where such results are to be found. In the graphic representation the experimental curves have been shown together with the corresponding calculated curves, which all are straight lines. In the calculation such activity coefficients as might be found in literature have not been taken into consideration. We have, therefore, discussed the activity relations of the substances and calculated the activity coefficients of such solutions of the substances in question as give freezing point depressions of 0.186°, 0.52°, and 0.93°. Furthermore we have compared our own activity coefficients with those of other authors. The result of the work is a proposal for a future Danish pharmacopoeia, and in this proposal all the experimental curves in figures 31—38 are drawn within the interval of 0° to 0.52°, which latter temperature is the freezing point of an isoosmotic solution. In these figures the congruent sodium chloride curve has also been drawn, so that it is easy to read from the figure how much sodium chloride must be added to a given hypotonic solution.

Finally a determination has been made of the vapour pressure of most of the solutions for parenteral use and the liquids for the treatment of tissues that are described in the Danish pharmacopoeia, the Dispensatorium Danicum, and the DAK, and where it has been possible, proposals have been given for alterations producing isoosmotic solutions.

9. *References.*

1. *Baldes, E. J.:* J. Scientif. Instruments *11*, 223, 1934.
2. *Blegen, E. M.:* Vanndiuresen. Bergen 1940.
3. British Pharmaceutical Codex. London 1934.
4. *Böhme, H.:* Archiv der Pharmazie *274*, 255, 1936.
5. *Collip, J. B.:* J. Biol. Chem. *42*, 207, 1920.
6. *Dreser, H.:* Arch. exp. Path. & Pharmak. *29*, 305, 1892.
7. Dispensatorium Danicum. København 1938.
8. *Eykman, C.:* Virshows Arch. *143*, 448, 1897.
9. *Hamburger, H. J.:* Zieglers Beitr. allgem. Path. & pathol. Anat. *14*, 443, 1893.
10. Handbook of Chemistry and Physics *21*, 1306, 1936—37.
11. *Heilbrunn, L. V.:* An Outline of General Physiology. Philadelphia & London 1937.
12. *Hill, A. V.:* Proc. Roy. Soc., London Ser. A. *127*, 9, 1930.
13. International Critical Tables *4*, 254, 1929.
14. *van Itallie, E. J.:* Jahresbericht der Pharmazie *53*, 196, 1918.
15. *Koeppe, H.:* Pfluegers Arch. *62*, 567, 1896.
16. *v. Koranyi, A.:* Z. klin. Med. *33*, 1, 1897.
17. *Krogh, A., Lund, C. G. & Pedersen-Bjergaard, K.:* Acta Physiolog. Scand. *10*, 88, 1945.
18. *Krönig & Fueth.:* Z. Geburtshilfe & Gynäk. *13*, 177, 1901.
19. *Landolt-Börnstein:* Physikalisch-chemische Tabellen.
    5. Auflage. Berlin 1923.
    5. Auflage, 1. Ergzbd. Berlin 1927.
    5. Auflage, 2. Ergzbd. Berlin 1931.
    5. Auflage, 3. Ergzbd. Berlin 1936.
20. *Lumiere, A. & Chevrotier, J.:* Bulletin des Sciences Pharmacologiques *20*, 711, 1913.
21. *Margaria, R.:* J. Physiol. *70*, 417, 1930.
22. *Nixon, W.:* The Pharm. Journ. *83*, 568, 1936.
23. Pharmacopoea Danica. København 1933.
24. Pharmacopoea Helvetica. Bern 1933.
25. Pharmacopoea Norvegica. Oslo 1939.
26. Remington's Practice of Pharmacy. Philadelphia & London 1936.
27. *Rosenthaler, L.:* Schweiz. Apotheker Zt. *78*, 85, 1940.
28. *Schou, S. A.:* Dansk Farmaceutisk Aarbog. København 1936.
29. *Stewart, G. N.:* J. Physiol. *24*, 219, 1899.
30. *Uteau & Saint-Martin:* Reference in the »Revue de Therapeutique Medico-Chirurgicale« *80*, 678, 1913.
31. *Veit, J.:* Z. Geburtsh. & Gynäk. *42*, 316, 1900.
32. *Viola, G.:* Riv. ven. sci. med. 18, 1901.
33. *Warburg, E.:* Compt. rend. du Lab. Carlsberg, Sér. chim. *22*, 547, 1937.
34. *Winther, J.:* Arch. Physiol. norm. Path. *8*, 114, 1896.

V. ABBREVIATIONS

In addition to the abbreviations in more general use the following are employed in this work.

‰	=	1/10 %.
% w/v	=	weight volume percent.
a	=	the inclination of the straight line in the logarithmic system.
f	=	the activity coefficient.
F	=	the freezing point depression in °C.
K	=	the concentration in ‰.
M	=	the molecular weight.
n	=	the number of ions in which a substance is dissociated in watery solution.
DAK	=	Danmarks Apotekerforenings Kompositionsudvalg 1944.
D.D.	=	Dispensatorium Danicum 1938.
F.n.c.h.	=	Formulae nosocomiorum civitatis havniensis 1922.
Ph. Dan.	=	Pharmacopoea Danica 1933.

VI. INDEX.

LATIN.

VII. INDEX.

ENGLISH.

Printed in Dunstable, United Kingdom

91221460R00098